The *Magical* MENOPAUSE DIET

DR. MARY DOUZJIAN PHARM. D.

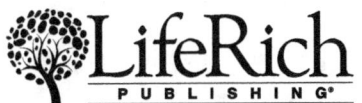

LifeRich Publishing is a registered trademark of The Reader's Digest Association, Inc.

LifeRich Publishing books may be ordered through booksellers or by contacting:

LifeRich Publishing
1663 Liberty Drive
Bloomington, IN 47403
www.liferichpublishing.com
1 (888) 238-8637

Interior Image Credit: Mary Douzjian

ISBN: 978-1-4897-2509-7 (sc)
ISBN: 978-1-4897-2508-0 (hc)
ISBN: 978-1-4897-2510-3 (e)

Library of Congress Control Number: 2019914928

Print information available on the last page.

LifeRich Publishing rev. date: 10/31/2019

Contents

Introduction

Disclaimer: Any reference to any individual in this book is purely fictitious and initials have been used in the stories at the end of the book, to illustrate certain disease states of appetite.

Any attempts to follow this diet must be endorsed by a personal physician, and the author is in no way liable for any outcomes due to individuals having adverse effects of following this diet.

The condition of our bodies is more important than ever. Our health is directly related to our weight. Working as a pharmacist, I deal with patients with many disease states that are worsened by weight gain.

This book is the story of how I came to gain weight after menopause. My doctor told me that it is common to gain ten to twenty pounds in perimenopause. I had always weighed 130 pounds, my ideal body weight, for the eight years after my marriage. Then I had my first son and gained 28 pounds, all of which I lost in the first 3 months after delivery, in conjunction with breastfeeding. This process was repeated 4 years later with my second son. So I became alarmed when 10 years into menopause I weighed in at 160 pounds, my full term pregnancy weight! I had gained ten to fifteen pounds when I stopped menstruating, as my doctor had predicted. I became used to weighing in between 140 to 145 pounds. I was still able to fit into my size 8, albeit a little tight.

Then my weight crept into the low 150's and I tried Weight Watchers, which did not work for me. I needed a diet with set parameters and not so many choices and variation in diet components. I also tried the chain weight loss centers, and lost 12 pounds, ending up in the low 140's again. Then I had the pattern of gaining 10 pounds again in a couple of years. I had actually stopped weighing myself, although I do own a scale. Shockingly, when I stepped on the scale, it registered at 160 again! I had recently been on a cruise and that had also contributed to sending me up to 160 again.

A trip to the Palm Desert gave me a week to relax, swim, run on the treadmill and think about losing weight. I realized at this point that a lifelong commitment was necessary[1]. I was the one teaching lifestyle changes to my patients. Now my life was about to change in the interest of my weight and health.

This book was also written in the interest of helping you, the reader.

I am going to achieve my goal weight of 130 pounds again and readers are invited on this journey with me. My height is 5ft 5ins, or 65 inches, and the ideal body weight for me is 130 pounds.

So many diet books talk about a particular diet, such as:

- South Beach diet [8]
- The Ketogenic diet
- The Paleo diet
- Weight Watchers
- Atkins for Life [1]
- Eat Right for Your Type [7]
- The Doctor's book of Food Remedies
- What to Eat When [11]
- Nutrisystem
- Jenny Craig
- Mayo Clinic Diet

- MediFast
- BistroMD

The above list names only a few of the myriad diets discoverable on Google. However there is no weight tracking to look at, day by day, in these diet books. Also there is not a lot of portion measurement in a most of those books, and a "slice of bread" can vary by 100 calories. There may be before and after pictures and total weight loss summaries, but not actual daily weights and the feelings that went along with the weigh in and weight loss.

If the diet supplies the meals, then the dieter may fail to learn the do's and don'ts of meal prep and shopping, and gain back the weight that was lost in the long run. The meal cards in this book are based on the one person who wants to be on that diet=YOU. You do not have to cook a meal or recipe and then decide how to split it into 4 portions, or be tempted to eat 2 portions, as it tastes so good!

Commitment is needed to learn the process of whole food diet eating and way of life.

A big part of the path ahead is to know what to expect in terms of time and weight loss. Unrealistic or dishonest claims may mean a dieter will give up after a month. I could have said I lost 16 pounds in the 1st month, but is that really what we want to do? So that is why I have included my weight tracking sheets for the length of time I was on the diet. There is also a space for notes on the tracking logs to document how one is feeling as the weeks go by, and events that may affect your weight loss, such as high days and holidays, weddings, anniversaries and birthdays. For instance, this diet does not include alcohol, but if you want to have a social glass of wine or champagne at a wedding, you can, and include it in your daily tracking of calories. You should be able to discern what 4-6 oz of wine looks like in the glass, and be able to sip slowly! Filling up the glass with 6oz of wine and gulping it down will only increase your blood sugar and alcohol levels quickly and lower your resistance to limit yourself to one glass only! If you have trouble, in the past, with aiming for sugar or alcohol highs, then politely say "no thank-you". You will need your full wits about you.

The chapter on the science of menopause outlines how our bodies need less calories as we age. There is also medical information and references on lower calorie diets resulting in lower disease rates, such as decreased morbidity and mortality, as well as increased longevity. As we lose weight and pounds our metabolic rate does decrease and our brain tries to trick us into eating more calories. That is why we have to have strict meal cards to stick to, to prevent losing our discipline.[12]

The meal cards used for this low calorie diet are simple but necessary. Every item eaten each day is written on the meal card, and so it is best planned a day ahead. All meals and snacks must be eaten and none skipped. The philosophy therein is to prevent grabbing items that have not been mapped out, and possibly cheating, due to hunger.

The stress in this diet is using mainly whole foods, no processed foods or sauces, so you will find no long, involved recipes in this book. The lovely thing about eating whole foods, is that once you have been shopping, there is not a whole lot of time spent on meal prep. Think of yourself as a hunter/gatherer in your kitchen, picking out the number of items for the day. Measuring accurately will ensure success on this magical menopause diet.

This diet book is written for busy professional women, whom work both in and out of the home. If the approach to weight loss is simple, then the easier is the successful outcome.

What is the philosophy of weight loss? We want to reach our beautiful shape and maximum health. Remember as we age we have to try a little harder to prevent weight gain by learning how to say no, and identifying diet saboteurs! You will find five stories at the end of the book, of types of diet failure, an illustration of how it can easily happen, if you are not prepared for it, and are not ready to nip temptation in the bud.

I love to exercise, but have little time in my weekly schedule. On my weekend off I try for one hour of walking or jogging, or 20 minutes on the treadmill on each of the weekend days. Then during the week I do weight lifting at the gym and have some weights around the house to use while watching TV. My yoga mat is left out in the living room and drop down on that for 10 minutes of stretches each day.

As a pharmacist, the importance of measuring accurately is always a concern. Cups, milliliters (mls), grams (gms), ounces (oz), teaspoons (tsp), tablespoons (tbsp.), are all used for measuring food and creating meals. In this book we will be using ounces rather than cups, and other inaccurate measuring devices.

Mandatory pantry auditing occurs at the beginning of the diet. Items to donate or dispose of are all processed foods such as cookies, food bars, chips, cakes, ice creams, American cheese, candy, soda and condiments and sauces. Diet soda such as diet cola, is not part of the diet as it can cause increased hunger. Large volumes of liquid at one time are not recommended due to potential for stomach swelling. Carbonated beverages such as Perrier may be sipped, in 4 ounce volumes. Wedges of lime, lemons and other fruits can be added to water to enhance the flavor. Stevia may be used to sweeten beverages. Teas and coffees are beneficial, but preferably without creamers that would add too much fat.

Last but not least there is information concerning the need for supplements, vitamins and minerals.

The exciting part of the journey for me was to find out how long it took to deflate the apple and reach the heaven of ideal body weight.

Ideal body weight for women: 45.5kg plus 2.3kg x each inch over 60 inches (5 ft)

Ideal body weight for me: 45.5kg + (2.3 x 5.5 inches)= 58kg=128lbs rounded to 130lbs

Goal is to go from 74kg to 60kg=14kg or 30 lb weight loss

Ideal body weight for men: 50kg plus 2.3kg x each inch over 60 inches (5ft)

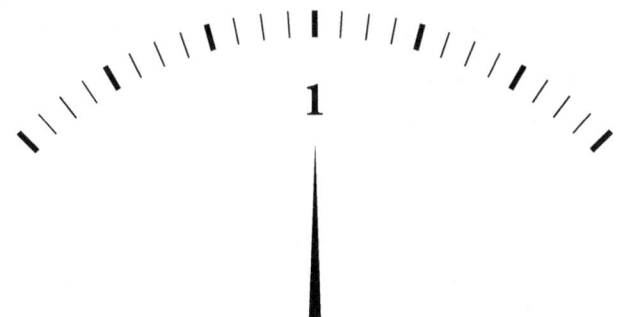

The Science of Menopause

Menopause can occur by the age of 50 in about 50% of women, and later in women with those genetics. Surgical menopause occurs when the ovaries are removed due to cancer or other causes. The pause of the menarche results in the ovaries ceasing to produce eggs each month, and the follicles no longer move down the fallopian tubes into the uterus. Menstruation ceases, and the shedding of the uterine wall no longer occurs. Most women are happy to say goodbye to the messy monthly period (the curse), but have to deal with other bodily changes such as night sweats, hot flashes from hormonal changes, as well as mood swings and weight gain.

Once estrogen levels decrease, chances of diseases increase, such as osteoporosis, changes in cholesterol levels and coronary complaints. Estrogen helps with the absorption of calcium into the bones and some women start to take hormone supplements to maintain estrogen levels. Others are unable to take estrogen supplements due to migraine headaches, cardiovascular disease or history of breast cancer. Diet is important to keep women feeling happy and well, low fat, high fiber foods and rich in antioxidants. Some dietary sources of phytoestrogens (estrogens made by plants) are almonds, cashews, apples, oats, wheat, corn, edamame beans and peanuts. Oats also contain beta glucan, a soluble fiber, as well as minerals such as potassium, magnesium, phosphorus, manganese, copper, and zinc. Soy based foods contain isoflavones, that may reduce menopausal symptoms, as Asian women eat more tofu, miso, edamame and soybeans and report less menopausal symptoms[4].

Calcium is needed during menopause, to avoid osteoporosis, so this diet includes low fat dairy such as reduced fat Swiss cheese, or Jarlsberg lite, low fat almond coconut milk, non-fat Greek yoghurt, greens such as spinach, legumes, almond milk and almonds. Pills of calcium citrate or calcium carbonate can be taken as a supplement to food intake, total 1200mg/day. There have been some studies that indicated excessive calcium intake can lead to calcification of the blood vessels and heart. Phosphoric acid may be a cause of aortic calcification and so no diet colas are allowed on the diet[5]. Vitamin D, 2000 units daily, is also helpful in preventing osteoporosis, and reducing falls.

Magnesium is needed to help with the calcium absorption into the bones, so do add a magnesium oxide supplement also, 400mg in the am and 400mg in the pm. Magnesium will also keep you regular, with the smaller portions on the diet menu. Magnesium will help with exercise, and heart and muscle function.

Mathematical observation of calories necessary for different age groups shows that as people age, the daily calories needed decrease for both sexes. Women, in particular, need fewer calories once in menopause.

The science of monthly blood loss shows up as a need for more calories in premenopausal women. Once in menopause women should eat less to maintain the same weight as from younger years.

Important calculation:

The calculation of 3500 calories per one pound weight loss is built into the diet. Seven days multiplied by 500 calories is 3500 calories, or one pound weight loss per week

So how do we determine our need for a day's worth of calories? I will use the BEE formula (basal energy expenditure), REE (resting energy expenditure) or the Harris-Benedict Equation.[17]

REE or BEE=655 + (9.6 x wt in kg) + (1.9 x ht in cm)-(6.8 x age)

Daily calories=655+(9.6x73kg)+(1.9x163)-(6.8 x 62)

=655+700+309-422=1242 calories/day

The above calculation is the basal energy needed for a day and can be multiplied by the factor of 1.2 or 1.3, depending on activity level. I chose to keep the basal calculation as women in menopause need fewer calories. The type of physique may also determine the quantity of calories, the more muscular body types will require more calories, while the higher the body fat percentage the lesser the amount of calories required.

To lose weight 500 calories is subtracted from the 1242, which is rounded to 700 calories per day. Each meal card contains meal plans for 500 calories per day, and this is due to the fact that one tends to under-calculate calorie counts. So in general, cutting 500 to 1000 calories from the daily intake will result in a 1-2 pound loss per week.

Most people want to lose weight quickly and are impatient to follow a diet. "This diet is taking forever", may be a common complaint. The reverse side of this coin is that weight lost quickly is regained quickly. The body takes time to readjust to the pounds lost, and will store extra calories taken in after the diet, to try to regain the former body weight.

It also takes the stomach time to shrink and adjust to smaller volumes of food. How often have you seen a friend lose 20 pounds in 3 months only to gain it all back? The body has not readjusted to the new weight yet. The dieter has reverted to a much higher intake of calories and the body captures those calories and restores the old fat deposits.[12]

So as you can see for the above calculations the body is designed for a weight loss of 4 pounds per month or 8 pounds per 2 months and so on. My goal is to lose 30 pounds to reach my ideal body weight, so I will be on the diet for as long as that takes. Additional weight loss will result from increasing exercise, for instance running on a treadmill for an hour will burn 300 to 350 calories. Doing that activity for 10 days will result in a loss of 1 pound!

So it will be important to maintain the diet for a length of time for the weight loss to be sufficient to maintain it. For instance, even if I was satisfied with a loss of 10 pounds and stopped, there could be a gain of 3 pounds as my body readjusts, leaving only a net loss of 7 pounds.

The basic metabolic rate (BMR) represents the minimum amount of energy expended in a fasting state, to keep a resting, awake body alive in a warm environment for a sedentary person, basal metabolism accounts for 60-70% of total energy use by the body.

For a 60kg woman use a BMR of 0.9kcal/kg per hour, so 60 x 0.9=54 kcal/hour.

So 54 x 24 =1296 kcal would be the calories needed for 24 hours. That amount of calories is general and will vary with age, a greater need for lean body mass and larger body surface area, male gender and caffeine and tobacco use. The amount of lean body mass a person has is the most important factor, and physical activity will help maintain muscle, and keep a high basal metabolic rate. The body may also shift into energy conservation in this low calorie diet, decreasing the BMR by about 10 to 20% or 150 to 300 calories/day. The BMR may also decrease by 1-2% for each decade of aging.

The thermic effect of food (TEF) occurs when the body uses energy to digest, absorb and further process the nutrients recently consumed. Food composition also affects the TEF, with protein using more digestive energy than carbohydrates or fat rich meals, because it takes more energy to convert amino acids into fat. Larger meals result in a higher TEF, than the same amount of food eaten over many hours.

As I want to lose 30 pounds I calculate that I would have to be on this diet for 30 weeks, losing a pound a week, or 7 to 8 months. This also seems like a good amount of time for my body to readjust to the lower weight. The weight loss should also be slow to allow the skin to shrink, as rapid weight loss can cause wrinkles and stretch marks. Eating smaller portions, as described in chapter 2, is crucial to the magical menopause diet. Ignoring portion size will result in decreased weight loss.

Fasting for a day is acceptable if tolerable per individual, better to experiment on a day off from work. I tolerate a day of fasting well, and actually feel better mentally as I don't use any energy to digest food. My metabolism is able to convert glycogen deposits, from the liver and fat stores from my abdomen, to keep my blood sugar level constant. Intermittent fasting or alternate day fasting(ADF) is also a good plan to get to goal if at a plateau.[12] Some may find it easier to fast for a day, and then eat normally the next day. I find it easier to have some food each day, but maybe eat all the 500 calories for breakfast and lunch and then not eat between 5pm and 9am the following day.(16 hours of fasting). The body will then use up all the glycogen in the liver and then start to pull lipids from body fat depots for further energy. It is better if that happens at night when asleep, as less hunger is felt, and it is normal for the body to deplete glycogen stores at night when the body is resting. Some of us will balk at this method, but then think of the opposite, continuously munching all day long, and punishing our system to digest and absorb all those calories! Sometimes a body just needs a rest, and that includes our teeth, tongue and jaw muscles! Some religions mandate days of fasting so that the mind is clearer to think of spiritual needs above physical needs. Spiritual strength will give the body increased reasons to become healthy.[13]

Intermittent fasting can have benefits that go beyond weight loss, including cardiac improvements and maintaining muscle mass. Fasting for short periods, within the day, say from 4pm to 8am the following day, is easier than fasting for several days. The 16 hour fast reduces insulin levels and as no food challenge is within the system. Night time is the best time to do the fasting, as glycogen is converted from the liver, into glucose in the bloodstream. We do not feel any pain!

We can enjoy a good breakfast and lunch and then fast overnight. The gut biome may also benefit from the rest. Over-challenging our GI systems with larger meals can lead to GERD (gastroesophageal reflux) and interrupt sleep. Remember that fasting does not include nibbling, which negates the metabolic purpose.

Exercise is extremely important for the mind and the body. Our sedentary lives today reduce the need for calories. We must set aside 20 minutes per day for some type of exercise or movement. Yoga, jogging, tai -chi, skipping rope, riding a bike or stationary bike, swimming or walking, all yield movement that is satisfying. Magically, endorphins are released, that improve our mood and well -being. Blood moving through our muscles, and lymph through our lymphatic-system, help clean the toxins from the tissues and organs, an added benefit of exercise. Chapter eight describes some helpful exercises and targets muscles that need to be worked during menopause in particular. The combination of a healthy diet and moderate exercise will aid us in our goal of losing unwanted pounds!

Some women in their later years have time to devote to sports, such as marathon running or extensive swimming. Most of us generally have time for moderate activity. Personally I find yoga rewarding, relieving stress by breathing deeply, keeping oxygen levels optimal, and improving blood circulation through the muscles and organs. Exercising harder and for longer periods may help break through a plateau, when weight loss seems to have come to a standstill. Yoga is good for both hypotensive individuals as well as hypertensive types, calming the nerves and returning blood flow to the heart and brain.

Exercise can also be a solution to food addictions. Instead of reaching for a candy bar, twenty minutes on the treadmill will be a mood improver. Women gain weight in menopause due to mood swings, hot flushes (drinking gallons of orange juice and soda), interrupted sleep (checking out the refrigerator at midnight) and changing body chemistry (trying various HRT, that could increase weight). It is crucial to find an exercise routine that is fun and gratifying and schedule times to perform. Sugar addiction is not the problem that nicotine and alcohol can be. However serotonin is released when sugar levels increase, increasing the feeling of calm and contentment. A person may love to have a bagel and cream cheese for breakfast, not knowing that their glycemic index is going through the roof! However their friends don't mind as that person's mood is pleasant. Exercising will increase endorphins but so will sugar intake. Break habits of eating unhealthy sugars containing corn syrup, and replace those snacks and processed foods with fresh fruit, which contains natural sugar called fructose. After a while the sweet cookies and especially candy will taste too sweet and synthetic, so stay with it and don't eat the addicting sweet foods that will never fill you up! Fruit contains fructose, but it is not concentrated, as in candy, and the fiber helps slow down the absorption of the fructose sugar. It would be extremely difficult to get any damage from eating fructose in whole fruit, while conversely high fructose corn syrup is a chemical and can cause inflammation in the body. Do not confuse the two, as whole fruits are beneficial, and loaded with other antioxidants and minerals. Do not drink from fruit juice concentrates, as fruit juice is NOT on the diet, only the whole fruits with the fiber.

Research shows that postmenopausal women have an increase in intraabdominal and trunk fat when compared to premenopausal women. The studies found that during early menopause, there is an increase in intraabdominal fat, the deeper visceral body fat. These changes were consistent among age and weight. An increase in intra-abdominal fat is linked to a higher risk of high blood pressure and myocardial infarction, diabetes and elevated cholesterol. Therefore the shift in body fat is more than a mere cosmetic issue.

The decline in hormones during and after menopause is just one part of the menopause belly. For many women their level of activity slows with age and many women do not reduce their calorie intake, to match the lowered activity level, coupled with a decreased muscle mass from less exercise, and lowers the metabolic rate leading to an increase in stored fat.

New exercise regimes should concentrate on the core, focus on the muscles that support the core, such as

- Front and side planks
- Reverse crunches
- Medicine ball twists
- Prostrate biking
- See the chapter devoted to exercise routine

Let's look at Menopause Myths:

- That the ovaries stop functioning and a women is infertile
- That a woman has estrogen deficiency and hence a hormone imbalance
- That a woman gains weight and her bones become brittle
- That ERT will correct the problems

In Fact

- A healthy women's ovaries function throughout her life and continue to produce hormones, and eggs,
- A women frequently has higher estrogen levels after her periods cease and there is no ideal balance to be disturbed
- Androgens which influence the libido or interest in sex, continue to be produced and in many women, tend to be higher after menopause
- Estrogen ERT can, at best, temporarily mask the symptoms blamed on menopause.

- At worst, by suppressing the ovary/ovarian activity, it can cause the ovary to atrophy, and also increase a woman's risk of cancer
- Healthy women taking ERT are subject to a higher risk of cancer of the uterine lining and breast cancer
- Binge eating is associated with decreased estradiol and increased progesterone

Estrogen also has anti-inflammatory properties and helps with the white blood cells or neutrophils.

So a little on biosynthesis, the estrogen is produced in the ovaries. FSH stimulates the ovarian production of estrogens by the granulosa cells of the ovarian follicles and corpus luteum, some by the liver, pancreas, bone, adrenal glands, skin, brain, adipose tissues and breasts, these secondary sources are important in post-menopausal women. The ovaries produce both estrogen and testosterone

Postmenopausal estrogen levels 7-40 pg/ml

Prepubescent females	8-29 pg/ml
Pubescent females	10-200 pg/ml
Premenopausal adult	17-200 pg/ml

The average woman will spend one third of her life in menopause, and the morbidities associated with treating menopausal symptoms must be investigated. 75% of menopausal women complain of vasomotor symptoms, such as hot flashes, anxiety, perspiration and palpitations and vulvovaginal symptoms, such as vaginal atrophy, dryness and itching, due to fluctuating estrogen levels.[14]

Conjugated estrogen, micronized estradiol, transdermal estradiol (patch), estradiol ring, combination estrogen-progestin, IM estrogen, depot estrogen, are forms of available estrogen. Standard low dose estrogen can reduce the symptoms as well as prevent postmenopausal hip, spinal, and non-spinal fractures.[16] Use of estrogen alone or in combination with a progestin was found to reduce symptom severity when compared with placebo. Estrogen only therapy is recommended for those without a uterus. Addition of a progestin is recommended in patients with a uterus, to prevent endometrial hyperplasia and potential endometrial cancer. The benefits that HRT have on bone density decrease rapidly after stopping therapy and FDA approval for prevention of OP for some products, does not include treatment of osteoporosis.

Major risks associated with the use of estrogen replacement include venous thromboembolism, ischemic stroke, increased incidence of endometrial cancer with estrogen without progestin, and increased risk of breast cancer when HRT is used beyond 3-5 years. Counseling points are to be aware of signs of pulmonary embolism, deep vein thrombosis, stroke and myocardial infarction.

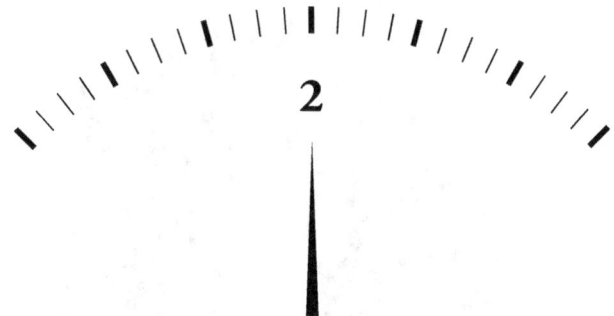

2

The Importance of Portion Measurements

The key to weight loss is to determine which liquid and solid measurements are going to be used in the diet and learn how to use those measuring tools.

We will use a food scale, pyrex measuring cups or jugs, tablespoon (tbsp.) and teaspoon (tsp), grams, millilitres (mls), ounces as measuring tools.

One teaspoon=5mls

One tablespoon=15mls

One ounce=30 grams (gm) or 30mls

One cup=8 ounces (oz) or 240mls (using the pyrex measuring jug has both mls and oz inscribed)

The picture below shows 4oz of bean salad or half cup or 8 tablespoons, the most accurate measurement would be in the pyrex jug. Check out the size of the teaspoon in relation to the bowl. You can practice by measuring 8 tablespoons into the jug to see if it reaches the half cup or 4oz line.

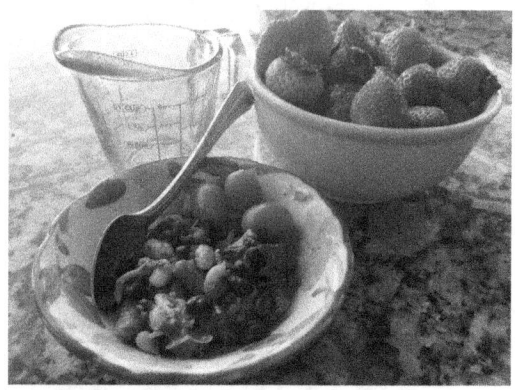

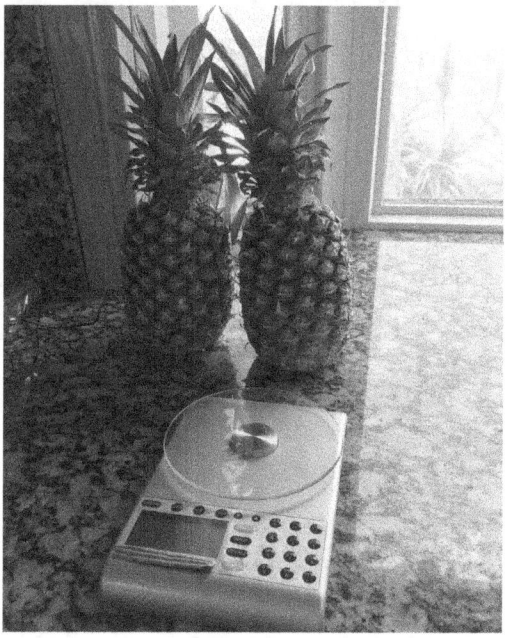

The food scale would be the most accurate, cover the plastic disk with wrap and measure the 4oz of bean salad on the scale. See how it compares to the amount measured in the pyrex jug and from the tablespoon measurements. Most likely the 8 tablespoons will over-measure the food portion.

When eating out it will be important to be able to eye ball the serving size, and only eat that amount.

Once you are familiar with measuring portions you will no longer have trouble losing weight.

Some hints:

Use a salad plate or small bowl to eat the meal

Avoid using large dinner plates as it may encourage you to take a larger serving.

Use whole foods as measurements, for example, one medium orange or apple, or half a medium banana

I prefer using the pyrex cup to measure servings of salads, vegetables and soups, rather than the palm of your hand, a deck of cards, a handful, a computer mouse, a cupcake wrapper, because it is easy to cheat by taking a huge handful rather than a small one! In other words all servings must have been measured and are quantifiable! Some of us have larger hands than others!

Measurement should be consistent.

When you are eating nuts, please see the calorie-protein listing, as these portions of nuts must be counted. I always laugh at the portions on the packet, about 4 servings, and then you count the amount in the packet, and it actually is a serving and a half. So be careful of calorie listings, as you may be eating 2-3 times the calories you think you are. Do not mindlessly eat the nuts out of the bottle or the bag, as it will be easy to overdo it. Take the nuts, count them into a bowl, and only then start to eat. Nuts are rich and delicious, and the flavors are natural, so we do not need to add extra salt, sugar or flavors. Remember that nuts are calorie dense. Mother Nature condensed the calories so that a tree could be started out of one of these pistachio, almond, cashew or walnuts! Have respect!

Nut trees have traditionally been owned by indigenous migratory tribes, who know when the nuts are expected, and come to claim their crop! Nuts had high food value in history for good reason.

N and N nibbled nicely on cashew nuts, as no carbs were noted on the nutrition information.

Remember nuts are mainly half fat/oil and half protein, fats have twice the calories of carbs, but the advantage is that nuts are crunchy, flavorful and full of healthy, unsaturated oils.

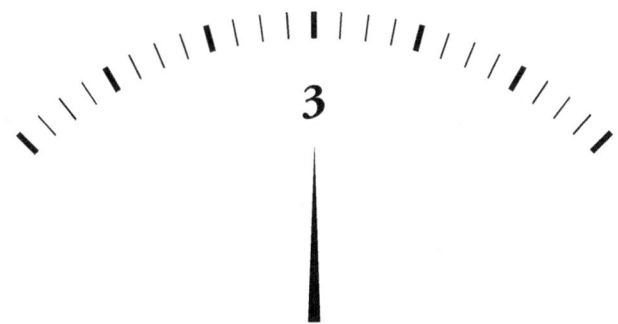

3

Ten Acceptable Food Groups/ Lists of Calories

It certainly pays to eat a good variety of foods as each food group contains valuable nutrients. We will be trying to eat only whole foods, so hopefully you have disposed of all processed foods in the refrigerator and pantry.

A quick discussion of the groups of carbohydrates, fats, proteins, fiber, minerals and vitamins will advise you of why these food groups are used in the diet.

Carbohydrates are needed in every diet and supply 4 calories per gram, about half of 1gm of fat, which is 9 calories. Complex carbohydrates are found in grains, breads, sweet potatoes, vegetables, corn, and beans. I did not mention pasta, because it is not a whole food and does not feature in this diet.

Simple carbohydrates-which are sugars-keep the energy levels up and the nervous system in gear. Fresh fruit, milk and honey are the healthy simple carbohydrates. The refined sugar found in soda, desserts, candy and processed foods and sauces, does not have any nutrients and is a junk food. Unfortunately we are raised on awful "treats" of candy bars and candy at every turn throughout the year, starting with Valentine's

Day, and then at Easter, Halloween, and Christmas. From the tender age of infancy we have been conditioned to the sickeningly sweet taste of corn syrup in most candy, cookies, bread and cakes. Cane sugar is not any better, increasing our blood sugar rapidly, and spoiling our appetite for real foods. Milk chocolate is loaded with sugar and one chocolate block/ nugget alone has 50 calories of antioxidants, but the sad truth is that it still loaded with sugar (And who can stop at just one?). Taking a tablespoon of cocoa and adding a packet of stevia and a tablespoon of evaporated milk will give you a relatively calorie free treat and antioxidants!

Fats are needed in bodily functions but we need to choose the beneficial types of fat to eat. The fat soluble vitamins are A, D, E, K [17]. Remember too much unhealthy saturated fat or hydrogenated fat will lead to heart disease, obesity, cancer, diabetes and atherosclerosis. Olive oil is a monounsaturated fat that lowers LDL and increases HDL cholesterol. Avocados and peanuts also contain unsaturated fats and contribute to a feeling of fullness. However, only small servings are advised as these foods are very calorie dense. One tablespoon of olive oil contains 120 calories, while one tablespoon of balsamic vinegar contains few calories, so mixing your own tasty salad dressing will add 120 calories to the salad or recipe. Fish oils contain omega-3 fatty acids that lower LDL cholesterol and triglyceride levels. The omega-3's also have an anti-inflammatory effect, and are important to lower atherosclerosis formed from high sugar levels in diabetes, and cholesterol.

Fiber is important in the diet, and intake should be 20 grams per day. The Magical Menopause Diet will include most fruits and vegetables available. We will not make a distinction between those that contain higher carb counts than others, as a varied intake will keep us occupied with different food tastes and textures, as well as antioxidants. That is the advantage of using a calorie count and not fussing over carbohydrates.

If you do decide to take a fasting day then you should take Benefiber three times that day to ensure proper waste removal though the GI tract.

Remember that fiber will increase energy burned to travel through the digestive tract as well as prevent colon cancer, diverticulosis and weight gain. Eating bulky foods help you to feel full as well as decrease the amount of food you will consume due the amount of chewing that is involved with eating salads, fruits and vegetables. After 20 minutes of food ingestion, your brain will start to let you know you can stop eating. In addition, all the other gobblers will have eaten all the food, so if you think you need a second helping of something, all the food will be gone!

Yes, it is true, Americans can consume the meal in 5-10 minutes, whereas the French may take up to 20 minutes to eat the same portion!

Pierre pondered points about the position of the poultry on his plate.

Proteins are the building blocks of the body and are used in growth and repair of cells, skin, muscles and bones. Our immune systems rely on proteins to manufacture our defense system, beta and T lymphocytes to fight against disease. The best sources of proteins are from meat, chicken, turkey, fish and dairy foods and contain all the essential amino acids. Legumes (beans, peas and peanuts) contain incomplete proteins but when combined with grains, nuts and vegetables will marry to provide complete proteins. Only 20 to 50 grams of protein are needed daily, so we will not be eating a high protein diet. I will add the protein content to the meal card to ensure that an adequate amount of protein is included, which should be over 20 grams for each card, as I will not add for all the vegetables, mainly the meat, cheese and nut components only. Proteins are metabolized into amino acids which take more digestive energy to convert into fats for storage, so are desirable in the diet for those trying to lose weight.

Top bloating food and beverages

- Carbonated beverages
- Onions, broccoli, beans, cabbage

- Soy products
- Foods high in fructose, apples, watermelon, cherries, pears
- Sugar substitutes such as sorbitol, mannitol, xylitol
- High fiber foods

Some are acceptable and others are not —eat as much cabbage as you can and you can fit in no chocolate!

As we are eating whole foods, food bars made out of soy protein are not acceptable. Food bars in general are NOT included on this diet, as it takes away from the practice of eating whole foods.

Lean cooked meats are better home cooked and then frozen in small portions, as these can be microwaved or defrosted overnight in the refrigerator. Store bought cold cuts can contain sodium nitrates which are a potential carcinogen. Store bought rotisserie chicken is a good choice, as long as not injected with oil, or basters.

1. FRESH WHOLE FRUITS
2. LEAN COOKED MEATS
3. TUNA FISH/SALMON/SHRIMP
4. EGGS
5. CHEESE/TOFU
6. FRESH/FROZEN VEGETABLES
7. ALMOND MIL/COCONUT MILK/2% MILK NON-FAT GREEK YOGHURT/2% COTTAGE CHEESE
8. NUTS-ALL SORTS, RAW OR ROASTED
9. BLACK TEA/GREEN TEA/LEMON-LIME WATER/ COCONUT WATER 6OZ/DAY
10. STEVIA/SOY SAUCE/TUMERIC/CURRY POWDER/ HERBS/BALSAMIC VINEGAR/OLIVE OIL/

CALORIE PROTEIN CALCIUM LISTING

FOOD	PORTION SIZE	CALORIES	PROTEIN GMS	CALCIUM MG
almonds	1oz -20 nuts	120	5	80
apple	one	60		11
asparagus	1 cup chopped	10		
avocado	half small	150		
bacon	2 strips	100	6	
banana small	one	100		0
bean salad	4 oz	100	6	60
bell pepper	half cup	20		
black beans	4oz	120	8	50
blueberries	20 berries	20		
bread one thin slice	one slice	100		
broccoli	4oz	50		70
cabbage	I cup chopped	20		30
cantaloupe	half cup	50		
carrots	half cup	40		
cashew nuts	20 nuts	100		10
cauliflower	1 cup chopped	20		20
celery	1 cup	20		
cheese low fat string	1 oz	80	6	200
cheese, mozzarella	I oz	100	8	200
cheese, parmesan	1 oz	100		330
cheese, s/Swiss reduced fat	21 gms-slice	50	7	200
chick peas	4oz	150	7	100
chicken breast	3 oz	150	20	20
collard greens	200gm	30		250
cottage cheese 2%	4 oz	100	12	100
cucumber	1 cup chopped	10		
edamame	3 oz	120	10	70
egg-boiled-poached egg	one	80	6	
feta cheese	1 oz	70	6	140
fish-smoked	2 oz	60	15	
grapefruit	half	50		
grapes	20 medium	100		

green beans	1 cup	30		40
ham	4oz	200	25	
hummus	4 tbsp	100	6	
kale	1 cup chopped	20		100
kiwi	one	50		60
Milk, almond coconut	8 oz	40	3	200
mushrooms	1 cup chopped	20		
oatmeal	4oz	100	3	
olive oil	1 tbsp/30 mls	120		
olives, Kalamata	10 large	60		
onions	half cup	20		
orange	one	50		40
papaya	3oz	60		20
Parmesan cheese	1 tbsp	20	3	50
parsley/tomatoes/cucumber	2 oz	20		
peach	one	30		
peanut butter	tbsp	100		
peas	4oz	100	5	25
pesto	1 tsp	50		
pineapple	half cup	40		
pistachio nuts	20 nuts	100	5	
pita bread	half small	75		
raisins	1 oz	100		
salmon burger	3 oz	170	20	180
salmon filet	4oz	200	24	200
sardines	3 oz	200	22	150
scallions	half cup	10		
shrimp	3 oz	100	15	70
spinach	1 cup	20		
steak	3 oz	180	25	15
tabouli salad(no bulgur)	4 oz	100		
tofu	4oz	50	10	200
tomato small	one	30		
Triscuit crackers	one	20		
tuna fish	3 oz	100	15	
turkey	4oz	200	25	

vegetable soup	8 oz	50		
walnuts	10 halves	120	3	30
watermelon	I cup chopped	50		
yoghurt, FAT FREE	8oz	100	13	350
yogurt, Greek FAT FREE	8oz	100	20	280

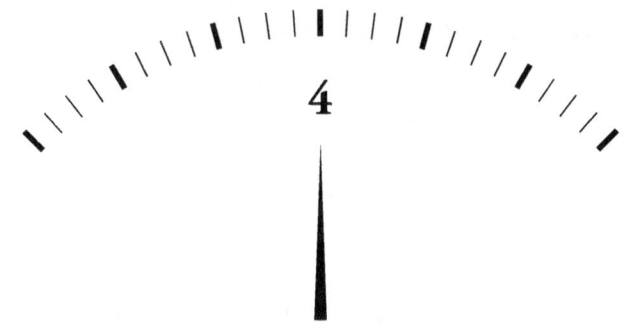

The Abyss Learning How
to Say No Thank-You

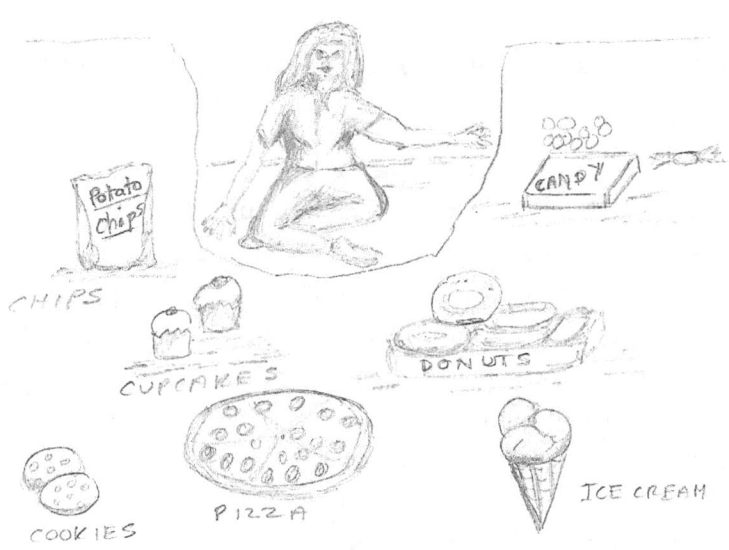

The illustration shows a person who is a slave to refined carbohydrates and sugars, supplementing their diet with cupcakes, cookies, candy, potato chips, donuts, and other processed junk. Refined carbs are low in fiber, vitamins and minerals and are linked to weight gain, and many serious diseases such as diabetes mellitus type 2. The fact that these foods do not satisfy, means that one can keep on eating until the whole bag is gone, and this problem may lead to eating disorders such as bulimia(overeating and vomiting), and anorexia (fear of even starting to eat)

There is really sometimes no other way out of the situation other than politely saying "No thank-you".

If you feel forced to elaborate, you can add you are on a diet, or that you are sensitive to salt or sugar.

The slave may be you or a friend. If it is you, your home should be clear of temptation. If you do break down and toss in a bag of corn chips while at the supermarket, open the bag and toss them all into the garbage when you get home, because that is where they belong!

Ten Ton Tessie tossed the chips tirelessly into the titanium truck trunk.

If your friend or family member is the culprit, and ignores your advice on mindless eating, and has open bags of junk food in the house, or work space, make sure you have some food item to counteract. My favorite is an apple or an apple cut into 4 quarters. Apples are whole foods, which remain fresh until cut into, and can take several hours to eat. Aim at eating one quarter every 15 mins and chewing slowly, so it will take up to an hour to consume the apple. If that does not have enough crunch value, then try tiny peeled carrots. Eat one to two carrots every 15 mins until you have consumed 4-8 carrots in the hour. You will amaze yourself at how tiny your bites can become!

Yes, and you can be proud that you have not clogged your GI system with low fiber, refined starches, hydrogenated fats and dangerous high fructose corn syrup, that may cause constipation and inflammation of blood vessels.

Remember to feel positive about your actions and do not feel left out due to peer pressure, namely because of the reasons discussed above.

Yes, I have stopped at the bakery on the way home, and bought almond croissants, macaroons and almond horns (my favorite). This treat was after achieving a goal loss of 15 lbs. However I was surprised to find that I was outraged at how sweet all the so-called treats were! I could only eat 1/8 of the pastry. My system had become attuned to the natural sweetness of fruit, and these artificial confections were an assault to my digestive system. The treats sat on a plate in the refrigerator for the next few days, until I decided I no longer wanted them, and they were stale, so I disposed of them.

Unfortunately I was taught as a child that candy, sweets and cakes, were a special treat after a meal, so I correlated that even as an adult. I suggest teaching your children that fruit, nuts and cheese and whole wheat crackers, or fresh berries stirred into low fat yoghurt, is the treat!

We find it easy to say "No thank-you" with some of the foods we don't like. I am not a big fan of sardines, so if someone offers me a slice of pizza with a sardine, they get an automatic "no thanks!"

If we view these refined carb creations as something that is negative for our digestion and health, then they also must get a mental or out loud no thank you also. Our microbiome can also change, when we are feeding bacteria with these refined carbs.

The addiction to sweet foods such as candies and cookies, can be partially reward and partly the serotonin response.

Your response to these types of foods must be to politely refuse any, or take only one piece, no more! Some cannot take only one chocolate or gummy bear and will keep eating until physically sick and the digestive process has ground to a halt. That is why only whole foods are allowed on this magical diet, and if you try to add anything extra to the spell, then it will lose its magical touch! Those large bags of corn chips and potato chips are NOT whole foods, please politely throw them into the trash, and those restaurants that offer free refills on the corn chips, just politely say NO! Just 5 large chips are 100 calories because they are fried, and also high in salt. No fried foods are allowed on this diet, and it will lose its magic if you try to change it.

Bulimia occurs because people can ingest large amounts of refined calories and then vomit them up once they regret eating them. This disease shows low will power in choosing correct foods and little respect for the human body and its functions. Eating correctly is a discipline that must be learned and strictly adhered to =no FUN foods. Guess what? These are no longer fun when they wind up on your hips or belly!

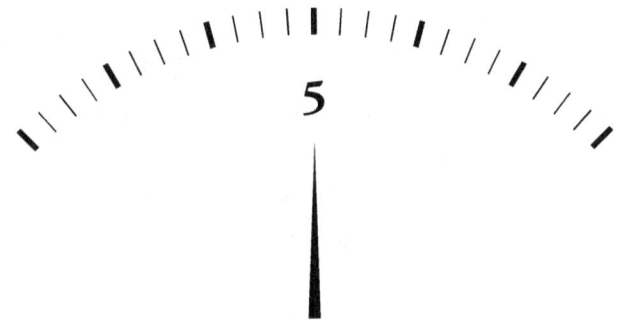

5

Weight trail sheets

These sheets are SUPER important to record the weight daily. I have listed my sheets to show mainly 2 things

1. Record and you will succeed
2. Do not record and you most likely will fail!

Discussion on the first sheet:

I was at my time share in the desert. I started to think about this diet and exercise every day, that being said I was lucky to lose the 3 POUNDS at the end of the 1st week, but as you can see from the calculation in the previous chapter, the 350 calories burned each day, used in jogging for the 5 days helped pull off the extra 2 pounds, without all the exercise I may just have lost my goal of 1lb (in subsequent weeks)

I had a good drop in the second week as I continued to use my diet cards and lost another 2 lbs, and at the 3rd week I had lost another 1.5 lbs for a total of 6.5lbs. Then it became harder to shift the weight, and I only lost 0.2 lbs at the 4th week, but I had been to a wedding, had some wine, and say no more!

Then I got busy and did not weigh myself for a week and did not write out my diet cards every day, and had no weight loss! The 6th week I weighed myself but had still not got back to writing the cards. The 7th week I tried an intermittent overnight fast from 4pm to 9am the following morning, and that seemed to help break the plateau, with a weight loss of 1.2 lbs for the 7th week. The 8th week showed a loss of 1.3 lbs for a total loss after 2 months of 10lbs!! My weight had changed from 161 to 151, better than my goal of 8lbs in the 8 weeks.

My next question is can I break into the 140's next week? Going into November, with Thanksgiving and the colder months, it was getting harder to work out. Also, I was travelling overseas for a family wedding at Christmas, and knew the travel would be disruptive to my diet.

So in the next 2 months of November and December I only succeed in losing 4.5 lbs, as I got sick just before leaving for New Zealand. I developed bronchitis and lost my voice, so am drinking lots of cough syrup and soups! But if I add the combined weight loss for the 4 months it totals 14.5 lbs or 2 stones, in the olde English measurements! I am feeling great and looking forward to losing another 16 pounds to reach my goal of 30 lbs. I am also buying new pants as my old ones are feeling rather too loose!

In the next 2 months of January and February I should be able to lose another 8 lbs as the weather will start to warm up and I can work out more, and then in March and April I will be in my final lap of the last 8 lbs to get to goal of 30 lb weight loss. See how planning works? No impulse here, I am right on target for the 8 months of weight loss September through April, and then the summer months of May, June, July and August to maintain!

My 4 weight trail cards follow with the condensed story of my diet.

__Mary muddled mightily with measurements to magnify the outcomes of the amazing diet!__

<div align="center">**<u>Weight Trail 1</u>**</div>					
date	weight	notes	date	weight	notes
9/14/2018	161	Ran on the treadmill	10/13/2018	Busy and	Did not
Did not weigh		Every day at the	10/14	Did not	write
Myself	on	Timeshare	10/15	weigh	Diet cards
Until weekend	Vacation		10/16		
			10/17		
			10/18		
9/21/18	157.8	Yeah!!	10/19	154	
1st week wt loss	3lbs	Goal: 3lbs	5th week wt loss	0 lbs	Goal: 1lb
9/22	157.5		10/20	weighed	Did not
9/23	157.2		10/21	But did	write
9/24	156.7		10/22	Not write	Diet cards
9/25	156.7		10/23	Down	
9/26	156.4		10/24		
9/27	155.8		10/25		
9/28			10/26	154	
2nd week wt loss	2 lbs	Goal: 1 lb	6th week wt loss	0 lbs	Goal: 1 lb
9/29	155.3		10/27	154	
9/30	155.2		10/28	154	
10/1	155.1		10/29	154	intermittent
10/2	154.9		10/30	154	fast
10/3	154.4		10/31	153	5pm /9am
10/4	154.3		11/1	153	To break
10/5	154.2		11/2	152.8	plateau
3rd week wt loss	1.5 lbs	Goal: 1 lb	7th week wt loss	1.2 lbs	Goal: 1 lb
10/6	154	Wedding	11/3	152.8	Continue to
10/7	155	weekend	11/4	152.7	Break thru t
10/8	154.7	Drank some wine	11/5	152.6	plateau
10/9	154.6	Ate more than	11/6	151.8	
10/10	154.3	usual	11/7	152	
10/11	154		11/8	151.5	
10/12	154		11/9	151.5	
4th week wt loss	0.2 lbs	Goal: 1 lb	8th week wt loss	1.3 lbs	Goal: 1lb

		Weight Trail 2			
date	weight	notes	date	weight	notes
11/10/2018	151.5	Wow/broke	12/8	148	
11/11	151.2	Thru to 150	12/9	148	
11/12	150.9	Can I get to	12/10	148	
11/13	150.4	140's this week?	12/11	148	
11/14	150.9		12/12	148	
11/15	150.8		12/13	147	
11/16	150.7		12/14	147	
9th week wt loss	0.8 lb	Goal: 150	13th week wt loss	1 lb	Goal: 147
11/17	150.6		12/15	146.5	
11/18	150.5	Yes!!	12/16	145.5	
11/19	150.4	Suddenly in	12/17	145.5	
11/20	149.3	The 140's	12/18	leave	Not able to
11/21	149.3		12/19	For NZ	weigh
11/22	Thanksgiving		12/20	gone	myself
11/23	150		12/21	Gone	
10th week wt loss	0.7 lb	Goal:149	14th week wt loss	Gone	goal
11/24	149.5	At the desert	12/22	Gone	Out of USA
11/25	149.4	again	12/23	Gone	
11/26	149.3	running	12/24	Gone	
11/27	149.2	treadmill	12/25	gone	
11/28	148.9		12/26	gone	
11/29	148.5		12/27	gone	
11/30	148.5		12/28	149	Return USA
11th wk wt loss	1.5 lbs	goal :148	15th week wt loss	2lbs	Gained
12/1	148.5	Maintain	12/29	148.5	
12/2	148	Weight	12/30	148.2	
12/3	148	Thru	12/31	148	
12/4	148	Holiday	1/1	148	New Years
12/5	148	parties	1/2	148	
12/6	148		1/3	148	
12/7	148		1/4	147	
12th week wt loss	0.5 lb	Goal: 147	16th week wt loss	2 LBS	Goal:147

			Weight Trail 3			
date	weight	notes	date	weight	notes
1/5/2019	147	Out of the	2/2	144	What kind of
1/6	147	holidays	2/3	144	birthday
1/7	146.7	Should be	2/4	143.9	Present
1/8	146.5	Easier to	2/5	143.2	Will I give
1/9	146.3	Lose now	2/6	143.9	Myself in 2019?
1/10	146		2/7	144	How many lbs
1/11	146		2/8	143.3	
17th week wt loss	1 lb	Goal: 146	21st week wt loss	0.7	Goal: 142
1/12	146		2/9	143.2	
1/13	146		2/10	143.1	Yes this is my
1/14	146		2/11	143	Birthday gift
1/15	146		2/12	143	Of 20 lbs
1/16	146		2/13	142.9	Weight loss
1/17	145		2/14	142.6	
1/18	145		2/15	142.7	My Birthday!
18th week wt loss	1	Goal: 145	22nd week wt loss	0.6	Goal: 141
1/19	145	Running this	2/16	144	Up a little
1/20	144	weekend	2/17	144	After a b-day
1/21	144.9		2/18	143	dinner
1/22	144.9		2/19	142	Weekend
1/23	144.7		2/20	142	Intermittent fast
1/24	144.5		2/21	141.8	
1/25	144.		2/22	141	
19th week wt loss	1	goal : 144	23rd week wt loss	1.7	Goal: 140
1/26	144		2/23	141	
1/27	144		2/24	140.9	Can I break into
1/28	144		2/25	140.8	The 130's?
1/29	143.9		2/26	140.7	
1/30	144		2/27	140.6	
1/31	144.4		2/28	140.5	
2/1	144		3/1	140.6	
20th week wt loss	0	Goal: 143	24th week wt loss	0.4	Goal: 139

Weight Trail 4					
date	weight	notes	date	weight	notes
3/2/2019	141.4	Still lagging	3/30	138.8	
3/3	141.3	By 1lb but	3/31	138.7	Not able
3/4	141.2	My goals	4/1	138.6	To get to the
3/5	141.1	Are pushing me	4/2	138.5	gym
3/6	140.9	ASH WEDNES.	4/3	138.4	
3/7	140.8	Into the 130's	4/3	138.4	
3/8	140.7	This week	4/5	138.3	
25th week wt loss	0.7	Goal: 140	29th wk wt loss	0.5	Goal:137
3/9	140.6		4/5	138.3	
3/10	140.5		4/7	138.2	
3/11	140.4		4/6	138.2	
3/12	140.3		4/9	138.1	
3/13	140.2		4/10	138	
3/14	140.1		4/11	138	Finally able to get
3/15	139.8		4/12	138	To the gym
26th week wt loss	1 lb	goal : 139	30th wk wt loss	0.3	Goal:137
3/16	139.7	Good that a	4/13	137.9	
3/17	139.6	1lb loss was	4/14	137.9	Walking in the desert again
3/18	139.5	achieved	4/15	137.9	
3/19	139.4	So not	4/16	137.8	Going to the gym
3/20	139.3	Slowing down!	4/17	137.7	
3/21	139.2		4/18	137.5	
3/22	139.1		4/19	137.4	
27th week wt loss	0.7	goal :138	31st wk wt loss	0.6	Goal: 137
3/23	139.1		4/20	137.3	
3/24	139.1		4/21	137.2	Easter
3/25	139.1		4/22	137.1	
3/26	139		4/23	137	
3/27	139		4/24	137	
3/28	139		4/25	136.5	
3/29	138.8		4/26	136.5	
28th week wt loss	0.3 lbs	Goal:137	32nd wk wt loss	1 lb	Goal: 136

Important comments:

As you can see from the weight trail sheets it is important not to miss a day to weigh in, it is gratifying to see the planning paying off! As I saw the blubber coming off, pound by pound, I was very happy and I felt great, in combination with my exercises I could feel I was improving my heart. I had better exercise tolerance and was happy with eating less.

I remember that growing up in Africa, as a teenager, I had begun to watch my weight. I had eaten smaller portions. Somewhere along the line I had started eating larger portions, maybe because I had two growing sons who were always hungry. When they were teenagers I always cooked dinner and probably started to eat more or bigger portions, or maybe eaten the leftovers? Also if we are eating a little more due to more socialization, then we need to hold the weight steady, even if it means intermittent fasting. I prefer to eat a little less at lunch and dinner rather than the intermittent fasting, because meals are a great time to spend time together and go over the day's activities and news.

The next chart on the diet cards will show you how to maintain the lower intake of calories through reducing portion sizes. As my stomach began to shrink, I did not want so much food, in fact when I went out for dinner I was satisfied with half the serving and took the remainder home for breakfast!

The body loses weight evenly, from fat deposits on the abdomen, arms and thighs, as well as the face and jowls. By losing a significant amount of weight, greater than 10 pounds, that effort will be reflected in the face, and the younger looking you will be looking back.

There are 4 weeks of diet cards prepared for you, or you can make your own. It is important to eat a variety of foods, but you will need to pick and plan for what you have in the house, and what you like, the shopping lists are also included.

Looking at the Weight trail 1, I lost 161-151=10lbs in the first 8 weeks. As I had suspected, the calorie reduction, resulted in a one pound/week weight loss, in conjunction with exercise. I also learnt that when I got lazy and did not use the diet cards I did not lose weight.

Looking at Weight trail 2, I broke into the 140's! It really makes a difference to titrate down to a 10 lb below number! However because this 2 month period included Thanksgiving, Christmas, New Year's and a major vacation, the weight loss was limited to 5lbs! I still view this as a success as weight gain is recorded for some during this holiday season.

Looking at Weight trail 3, I lost 7 pounds during this 8 week period, and was pleased with that amount. I gave myself a great birthday gift being in the low 140's!

Looking at the Weight trail 4, I broke into the 130's. I had not seen this weight figure since pre-menopause years! I lost 5lbs during this eight week trail as my body took some time to register the much lower abdominal fat content.

I have also started attending yoga class again at my gym. The lower body weight has given me much greater flexibility. The stress relief was advantageous, as I am a type A, and want to do everything now, if not sooner. Yoga slows me down and helps with my breathing.

Strangely though, I still feel as if I have excess belly fat! My body is built so all excess fat goes to the belly, while I have smaller buttocks and thighs. The Golden rule of course is never to miss weighing myself, preferably not even for one day.

Remember Scarlett O'Hara in Gone with the Wind? She had a 22 inch waist line. Her nanny made her fill up on yams before attending neighborhood parties. She really was full when she said she could not eat anything! Nanny did not want her making a pig of herself in front of the young men. She had her custom of eating before the party and very little at the party!

The stomach was engineered to be partially full when we were food gatherers, not bloated. If there was abundance it was taken back to the cave to be eaten later. Some nomadic bush cultures in South Africa would eat until bloated, only because they had to finish the kill, before scavengers arrived. Their physique took a beating because of the pattern of stretching their stomachs to capacity and then storing the excess calories as fat.

Personally I do not patronize buffets, preferring to only order a favorite starter at some restaurants. If dealing with a large portion of food for dinner, only eat half and ask for a doggy bag, even if you turn out to be the dog at breakfast!

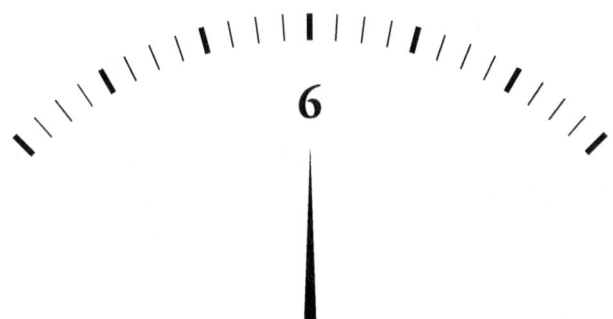

6

The Value of Meal Cards

Meal cards are an essential asset to improving your health and life through good eating practices. Eating the majority of calories before 5pm aids and can result in weight loss. As the majority of workers leave the house early in the day, the meal prep should be done the preceding day or the night before. Once our mindset changes we do not come home and expect to consume a large, calorie laden meal. We busy ourselves collecting food items for the next day, maybe putting salad materials in a container with some chicken breast, or a serving of tuna, and adding a serving of nuts and fruit. These items will be eaten for lunch and snack before 5pm. The following day's breakfast can also be made, by boiling eggs, or placing a measure of yogurt and fruit in a container. Coming home to prepare the food will be meaningful. We are reaping the benefits of even calorie intake during the day, and when night arrives we are not really hungry. We sleep better because our blood is pumping evenly through our body, including our brain, and not all congested around the GI area.

If we forget to take food to work with us, it is only acceptable to eat 250 calories after 5pm, it is not acceptable to eat all the days calories when returning home, hopefully the meal cards are valuable in that message! A day of intermittent fasting is acceptable if we are not feeling hungry at night.

Protein early in the day idea, helps to jump start the metabolism and keeps us full longer than carbs.

The nut snacks are filled with lysine and arginine and help reduce anxiety! Yes, working long hours can induce FAT-igue or fatigue, either way we are not giving in to eating candy. Some foods can lie to us through their looks, and that is why we must carry the diet card for the day with us and STICK to it, or stick it on our forehead!

You should eat all the food on the meal card, if you want to add some extra calories, that is up to you.

Tear out the blank or sample meal card and copy it, if you want to create your own meal cards, using a different combo of meals, according to your dietary needs. If you do skip a meal for any reason, you should keep Benefiber around the house, so that you do not get constipated. I am also recommending magnesium sulfate 250mg to 400 mg in the am and pm, to regulate bowel health, due to decreased food volume intake.

Do not let others intimidate you into ditching the diet card, those and weighing yourself EVERY day is an essential practice to be successful in weight loss over time, and then maintaining the weight loss.

DATE Day 1	FOOD ITEMS	CALORIE COUNT	
Breakfast	Half a pita	75	
	Boiled egg	60	6
	20 blueberries	30	
Lunch	Mixed green salad 2 cups		
	4oz of chicken breast/leg/thigh	200	20
Dinner	2 mandarins	60	
Snack	10 cashews	50	
TOTAL		~500	

NOTES: Eating the bulk of the calories before 5pm will help with weight loss. Try not to eat 3 hours before retiring for the night. The calories are listed on the right and the grams of protein far right.

Everything has a quantity listed, nothing is free, as eating too much salad overfills the stomach, and if adding a little salad dressing, may add extra calories, I advise using lemon juice, lime juice, wine vinegar, and if you must, some olive oil. Remember a tablespoon of olive oil is 120 calories.

DATE Day 2	FOOD ITEMS	CALORIE COUNT	
Breakfast	4oz of low fat cottage che ese	100	12
	1 small banana	100	
Lunch	Hummus 4 tbsp (recipe provided)	100	6
	5 pita chips	50	
Dinner	2 cups of mixed greens, one tomato, half a small cucumber	40	
Snack	10 walnut halves	100	
TOTAL		~500	

DATE DAY 3	FOOD ITEMS	CALORIE COUNT	
Breakfast	4oz of non-fat Greek yoghurt	50	11
	8 strawberries	20	
Lunch	2 cups of mixed cabbage/lettuce/spinach greens	20	
	4 oz of chicken breast	200	
Dinner	One orange	50	
	3oz tuna fish in water	100	15
Snack	20 pistachio nuts	100	
TOTAL		~500	

NOTES: Sweetened yoghurt available commercially is full of syrup and additives, stick to plain non-fat yoghurt and add your own sweet fruit, if not sweet enough add a packet of stevia.

The eggs and cheese for breakfast make for a filling and satisfying flavor, saving the carbs for lunch, with the pita bread and tuna fish.

DATE Day 4	FOOD ITEMS	CALORIE COUNT	
Breakfast	1 slice of lo- fat Jarlsberg lite cheese	50	
	2 sunny side up eggs/spray of Pam	160	12
Lunch	Half pita	75	
	Tuna fish 3oz(in water)	100	20
Dinner	Mixed green salad 2 cups with 10 kalamata olives	50	
	7 cherry tomatoes	20	
Snack	7 walnut halves	50	
TOTAL		~500	

DATE DAY 5	FOOD ITEMS	CALORIE COUNT	
Breakfast	Half grapefruit	50	
	4oz almond milk	50	
Lunch	Spinach salad with 8 mushrooms (raw or roasted)	20	
	3oz of grilled salmon	200	20
Dinner	7 medium shrimp grilled on skewers (sprinkle with curry powder)	120	15
	6 cherry tomatoes	20	
Snack	One small apple	50	
TOTAL		~500	

NOTES: the menus that are higher in protein will keep you feeling full, and the numbers in the column on the right are approximate grams of protein. There is some protein in the vegetables, but the amounts are insignificant in comparison with the lean proteins such as fish, chicken and dairy products.

Use the pyrex jug to measure the 6OZ of mixed fruit, you will be surprised how small the serving is.

DATE DAY 6	FOOD ITEMS	CALORIE COUNT	
Breakfast	6oz of mixed fruit salad watermelon/ cantaloupe/pineapple	150	
Lunch	3oz of turkey or chicken	170	15
	Half small roasted sweet potato	150	
Dinner	One tablespoon peanut butter	100	5
	7 celery sticks		
Snack	Half small apple	30	
TOTAL		~500	

DATE Day 7	FOOD ITEMS	CALORIE COUNT	
Breakfast	Half cup oatmeal	100	
	4oz of almond/coconut milk	50	
Lunch	Cucumber salad (one small cucumber peeled and sliced)		
	Half small avocado	150	
Dinner	Chicken vegetable soup 8OZ (see recipe)	150	10
Snack	7 walnuts	50	
TOTAL			

NOTES: Oatmeal is full of soluble fiber, as are the fruits, and that helps to keep the stomach full, and help pass waste regularly.

DATE Day 8	FOOD ITEMS	CALORIE COUNT	
Breakfast	one orange, half banana	100	
	4 oz. non-fat yoghurt	50	7
Lunch	Half pita pizza, 1oz low fat mozzarella cheese, 6 black olives		
	Scallions, one tomato sliced, all baked	200	7
Dinner	4oz of tabouli salad (no bulgur)(recipe provided)	50	
	3oz of smoked ono/salmon	100	15
Snack	6 small carrots	20	
TOTAL		~500	

DATE Day 9	FOOD ITEMS	CALORIE COUNT	
Breakfast	2 slices of grilled bacon	100	6
	One slice of reduced fat Swiss	50	
	3 triscuits (place bacon and Swiss on triscuits)	60	
Lunch	4 tbsp. hummus	100	6
	6 small carrots		
Dinner	Salmon burger	170	17
	1 tsp pesto	30	
	4 oz of tabouli	50	
		.	
Snack	One tomato	20	
TOTAL		~500	

NOTES: Triscuit crackers provide a need for the crunch factor, and at only 20 calories each, can be combined with cheese, smoked fish, and vegetables to provide flavor. The whole grain wheat will give some carb charge also. Goat cheese with fruit preserves has a savory/sweet turn to it also.

DATE Day 10	FOOD ITEMS	CALORIE COUNT	
Breakfast	4oz of cooked oatmeal	100	
	5 walnuts	50	
	Half small banana	50	
Lunch	4oz low fat cottage cheese	100	12
	Half apple	50	
Dinner	Mixed salad with spring greens		
	3oz of tuna fish	100	15
Snack	10 almonds	50	
TOTAL		~500	

DATE Day 11	FOOD ITEMS	CALORIE COUNT	
Breakfast	One small apple or half large apple	60	
	10 almonds	50	
Lunch	2 cups of mixed salad/8 black olives	20	
	3 oz of salmon/or tuna fish	150	15
Dinner	Chicken vegetable soup with 4oz of chicken meat		
	(Chicken broth with celery, carrots,)	150	20
Snack	One slice of low fat Swiss cheese	50	
TOTAL		~500	

NOTES: Fruit breakfasts give a flavor lift in the morning and nuts have a sustaining nature due to the fat and protein content. The salad and protein at lunch is a filling combination, and stops the carb slump that occurs with a sandwich.

DATE Day 12	FOOD ITEMS	CALORIE COUNT	
Breakfast	4oz of cooked oatmeal	100	
	5 walnuts halves/10 raisins	75	
Lunch	8oz cooked broccoli	50	
	1 oz of melted low fat Jarlsberg lite	50	7
Dinner	3oz of grilled steak	180	25
	One chopped tomato/one quarter grilled sweet onion	20	
Snack	6 celery sticks		
TOTAL		~500	

DATE Day 13	FOOD ITEMS	CALORIE COUNT	
Breakfast	2 egg omelette/one chopped tomato	200	12
	2 tablespoons of parmesan cheese	40	6
Lunch	One small apple		
	One tablespoon of natural peanut butter	100	3
Dinner	Baby spinach salad with wild salmon burger	170	25
Snack	10 raw almonds	50	
TOTAL		~500	

NOTES: Eggs can be used with the yolk or using the egg white alone and other zero vegetables can be added instead of tomatoes, like scallions, broccoli, red pepper, mushrooms and olives. Use only Pam or olive oil spray when coating the pan. Salmon burgers are easy to grill and full of oils that produce anti-inflammatory benefits.

DATE Day 14	FOOD ITEMS	CALORIE COUNT	
Breakfast	Fat free Yoghurt 8oz	100	13
	Half pear	30	
Lunch	4 triscuit crackers	80	
	2 oz smoked salmon	50	
	1 tbsp pesto	30	
Dinner	7 large grilled shrimp skewers	100	10
	6 mushrooms		
Snack	15 baby carrots	20	
TOTAL		~500	

DATE Day 15	FOOD ITEMS	CALORIE COUNT	
Breakfast	4oz cooked oatmeal with cinnamon	100	
	4oz coconut milk	50	
Lunch	One boiled egg	80	6
	One slice of low fat Jarlsberg lite	50	7
Dinner	Mixed bean salad (see recipe) 8oz	200	12
Snack	One tomato		
TOTAL		~500	

NOTES: Beans contain vegetable protein and are a great addition for those who want a non-animal source of protein. The benefit of plant protein is that it comes with a good fiber boost. If you are sensitive to beans, use green beans with diced red pepper, and skip the pinto beans and chick peas.

DATE Day 16	FOOD ITEMS	CALORIE COUNT	
Breakfast	One thin slice of toast with one tsp of jam	100	
	One slice of reduced fat Jarlsberg lite	50	7
Lunch	2 cups of iceberg lettuce/6 black olives		
	Half a small cucumber, one tomato		
	Two tbsp. feta crumbles or 1 oz feta cheese	100	5
Dinner	20 almonds	100	5
	20 small grapes/10 large grapes	100	
Snack	one orange	50	
TOTAL		~500	

DATE Day 17	FOOD ITEMS	CALORIE COUNT	
Breakfast	8oz of Greek yoghurt with half banana	100	20
Lunch	2 cups of chopped cabbage with 1 tbsp of olive oil,	150	
	One tbsp. of lemon juice, salt pepper		
	One chopped tomato or shredded carrot		
Dinner	3 oz of grilled steak	150	20
	4oz of blanched peas	100	
Snack	One peach or mandarin	30	
TOTAL		~500	

NOTES: Cabbage is a cruciferous vegetable that has a high percentage of fiber, and can be used with olive oil, for a vegetarian dish. The olive oil contains monounsaturated fat, protective against the atherosclerotic damage that saturated fats, such as butter and cream, can cause.

DATE Day 18	FOOD ITEMS	CALORIE COUNT	
Breakfast	One small banana or half a large	50	
Lunch	Half pita stuffed with iceberg lettuce	75	
	3 oz of chicken	150	15
Dinner	4 triscuit crackers	80	
	Slices of tomato		
	1oz of reduced fat mozzarella cheese	100	8
Snack	20 pistachios	100	5
TOTAL		~500	

DATE Day 19	FOOD ITEMS	CALORIE COUNT	
Breakfast	Half bagel with 1oz ham	150	15
	One slice of melted Jarlsberg lite cheese	50	10
Lunch	2 cups of mixed salad greens, radicchio, lettuce		
	3 oz of tuna fish /squeeze of lemon	100	15
Dinner	Vegetable soup with carrots, spinach, chick peas, onion	100	
Snack	One small apple	50	
TOTAL		~500	

NOTES: I know someone who loves bagels, but a whole bagel is too much for the glycemic index, so eat half a toasted bagel and add ham and low fat cheese to reduce the insult to the glycemic index! The other half bagel can be frozen for a repeat appointment!

DATE Day 20	FOOD ITEMS	CALORIE COUNT	
Breakfast	8oz fat free yoghurt	100	13
	Half chopped apple		
Lunch	Half a pita	75	
	Boiled egg/one tomato	80	6
Dinner	3oz tuna fish	100	15
	Assortment of lettuce/spinach salad 2 cups	10	
	One teaspoon olive oil/one tablespoon of balsamic vinegar	50	
Snack	10 walnut halves	100	
TOTAL		~500	

DATE Day 21	FOOD ITEMS	CALORIE COUNT	
Breakfast	One slice of low fat Jarlsberg lite	50	6
	Half a pita with one egg	150	6
Lunch	2 cups of mixed cabbage/carrot slaw	20	
	3 oz of chicken breast	150	15
Dinner	8oz of chicken vegetable soup	100	
Snack	One small pear	50	
TOTAL		~500	

NOTES: For those who cannot eat cheese due to a lactose allergy, the diet card below is cheese free and contains some calcium in the broccoli and salmon(see calcium table) romaine, kale, almond-coconut milk (buy the one with 50% of daily calcium added). You could also substitute hummus for the cheese selections as chick peas have high calcium content.

Avocadoes are high in calories, but provide the richness that increases the feeling of fullness and contain healthy monounsaturated oils/fats. Wild salmon burgers contain fish oils that are beneficial and lots of protein.

DATE Day 22	FOOD ITEMS	CALORIE COUNT	
Breakfast	Half cup of oatmeal	100	
	4oz of almond-coconut milk	50	
Lunch	2 cups of mixed salad greens (romaine lettuce and kale)	100	
	Tomato/quarter avocado		
Dinner	Salmon burger	170	20
	6oz of broccoli	50	
Snack	2 mandarins or one orange	50	
TOTAL		~500	

DATE Day 23	FOOD ITEMS	CALORIE COUNT	
Breakfast	3 oz grilled steak/lean hamburger	180	20
	Grilled tomato	20	
Lunch	6oz cooked broccoli/cauliflower	50	
	1 oz of low fat mozzarella	50	6
Dinner	2 cups of mixed slaw/cabbage/kale		
	Tsp of olive oil/one tablespoon balsamic vinegar	80	
Snack	18 almonds	100	5
TOTAL		~500	

NOTES: Red meat is the best source of iron for anemic people, and absorption is better than from vegetables such as spinach. Red meat once a week is a healthy choice.

DATE Day 24	FOOD ITEMS	CALORIE COUNT	
Breakfast	Half a small banana/1/2 orange	100	
Lunch	4 oz of grilled sea bass	150	20
	Arugula/red onion salad		
Dinner	4 triscuits/1oz goat cheese	180	8
	2 tablsp. Pure fruit jam or strawberry pure		
	(no corn syrup)		
Snack	20 raisins	50	
TOTAL		~500	

DATE Day 25	FOOD ITEMS	CALORIE COUNT	
Breakfast	Half a pita with boiled egg	150	6
	One slice of ham/one tomato	30	
Lunch	Hummus 4 tbsp.	100	6
	Chopped cucumber with 1 tsp of rice vinegar		
Dinner	3oz of chicken breast or leg	150	20
	2 cups of kale salad		
	One tsp olive oil/one tbsp. balsamic vinegar	50	
Snack	6 sticks of celery		
TOTAL		~500	

NOTES: A chocolate treat can be concocted from almond-coconut milk, cocoa and stevia, with hardly any carbs or fat! Enjoy!

DATE Day 26	FOOD ITEMS	CALORIE COUNT	
Breakfast	4oz low fat cottage cheese	100	12
	6 strawberries	20	
Lunch	2 cups mixed lettuce/spinach salad		
	Tuna fish 3oz	100	20
Dinner	8 medium shrimp grilled	140	17
	6 cherry tomatoes	20	
Snack	8oz of almond coconut milk	50	
	One heaped teaspoon of cocoa/stevia		
TOTAL		~500	

DATE Day 27	FOOD ITEMS	CALORIE COUNT	
Breakfast	2 egg omelete with 2tbs. parmesan cheese	200	15
	2 tbsp. chopped onion or scallions		
Lunch	One small apple	60	
	One tablespoon natural peanut butter	100	3
Dinner	2 cups of kale/lettuce salad with tomato and cucumber		
	1 tsp. olive oil and 1tbsp of balsamic vinegar	100	
Snack	15 small carrots	40	
TOTAL		~500	

NOTES: Omelets are weekend friendly foods, and can be low calorie when using free oil sprays, instead of butter or oil in the pan, adding high flavor foods such as onions and cheeses can give the omelet a lovely flavor. After cooking for breakfast, the lunch and dinner are easy prep! Chopped and washed salad in the bag is a no-brainer!

DATE Day 28	FOOD ITEMS	CALORIE COUNT	
Breakfast	Fat free yoghurt 8oz	100	13
	Half a pear	30	
Lunch	Mixed bean salad 8oz	200	12
Dinner	One boiled egg	80	6
	One slice of lean ham	25	
Snack	10 cashew nuts	50	
TOTAL		~500	

DATE Day	FOOD ITEMS	CALORIE COUNT
Breakfast		
Lunch		
Dinner		
Snack		
TOTAL		

NOTES: Blank diet card to copy and mix menus of choice

DATE Day	FOOD ITEMS	CALORIE COUNT
Breakfast		
Lunch		
Dinner		
Snack		
TOTAL		

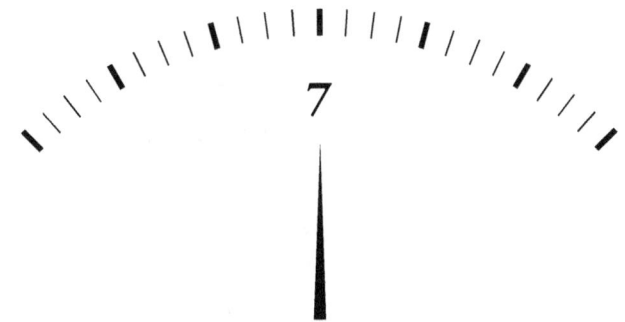

7

Shopping Lists for food variety, for the week or month

These samples shopping lists are prepared from the Meal Cards for your convenience.

The lists are in alphabetical order for an easy search, rather than fruit/meat/cheese.

Economical prices can be obtained in warehouse outlets on more expensive items such as nuts, meats and cheeses. Some non-perishable items are listed for the month and other perishables such as salad and fruits are listed for a week supply.

The list is not all inclusive and any items listed in the calorie listing sheet may be added.

Almonds	8oz bag (raw not roasted)
Apples	3 apples
Avocado	one small
Bacon	4oz package
Bananas	4 small
Beans, black	1 can

Beans, green	1 can
Blueberries	small container
Broccoli	one package, frozen
Cabbage	one small, or chopped in a bag
Carrots	8oz package/peeled baby
Cashew nuts	8oz bag (salted or unsalted)
Cauliflower	one package, frozen
Celery	one bunch
Cheese, lo fat mozzarella	one pound
Cheese, parmesan	8 oz, grated
Cheese, Jarlsberg lite	one pound
Cheese, Feta	8 oz
Chick peas	one can
Chicken breast	one pound, cut into 4 portions
Chicken, rotisserie	one, divide into 3-4oz portions
Cottage cheese 2%	one pound
Cucumber	one large or 4 small
Edamame	one bag in the pod
Fish, smoked	smallest package, or 3oz
Eggs	one dozen
Grapes	20 -40 medium
Ham, lean sliced	4oz
Hummus	8oz
Kale	one bag chopped and washed
Lettuce	one bag, mixed, washed
Milk, almond coconut	2 quarts
Mushrooms, canned	2 small cans
Oatmeal	one pound
Olive oil	8oz
Olives, Kalamata	one pound or 16 oz
Oranges	3 medium
Parsley	2 bunches

Peanut butter, natural	small container
Peas	8oz frozen
Pesto	small container
Pineapple	one small container
Pistachio nuts	one bag, in the shell (contains 100-200 nuts)
Pita bread (6 inch in diameter)	bag of six, or can buy more and freeze
Raisins	one oz boxes
Salmon burger	wild, one bag
Salmon filet	8oz (4oz portions)
Scallions	one bunch
Shrimp, medium	8oz (divided into portions of 6-7 shrimp
Spinach salad	one bag, washed
Steak	8oz (divided into 4oz portions)
Strawberries	one package
Tomatoes	6 vine ripened, box of cherry,
Triscuit crackers, original	one box
Tuna fish	assortment of 3 oz cans/packages or 5 oz cans
Walnuts	8oz package
Watermelon	one small container
Yoghurt, non-fat	16 oz
Yoghurt, Greek non-fat	16 oz

8

Movement Exercise and Toning

We should be proud of our bodies and our shape. The food we put in our mouths should be due only to hunger, and to fuel our bodies for proper health and action. Somewhere along the line our messages can get crossed, and we start to eat out of frustration, anxiety or boredom. We sometimes need to analyze the day to ensure we are spending some times on pure physical exercise.

There are basic through advanced exercises to banish the belly, butt and thighs. I have illustrated 12 exercises that I like and are relatively easy to perform. The amount of time and pace used or number of reps is up to you, the harder you work the greater the effect and results.

The first six exercises can be done using a yoga mat on the floor. The subsequent exercises should be performed at the gym.

1. The Crossover Crunch:

This uses opposite elbow to opposite knee and exercises the core, in particular the stomach muscles: the rectus abdominis. A modified version is to rest the ankle on the thigh and go elbow to knee. The point is to stress the stomach area and not the back or neck area.

Lie supine on the floor with your knees bent and hands behind your head, shifting your legs off the floor. Lift your shoulder blades off the floor and twist from your ribs to bring opposite elbow to knee, straightening out the leg and try 10 reps to start, and building on that as tolerated.

2. The Piriformis Stretch:

This exercise is also for the core and is wonderful if you suffer from back pain, especially if you spend all day typing on a lap top or computer key board. The piriformis and quadratus muscles are used.

Lie on the yoga mat and bring your left ankle over your right knee, as per diagram. Place both hands behind the right thigh, and gently pull towards your chest, until you feel the stretch in your buttocks. Hold for 15 seconds and then switch sides. Repeat the sequence with your right leg over your left thigh.

3. The Pointer:

Another core exercise helps develop and stretch the adductor magnus, obliques, rectus abdominus, and overall tones the legs, arms and abdominals. Begin on your hands and knees with your wrists below your shoulders, gaze at the floor keeping your head in a neutral position. Slowly slide the left leg backwards and then lift it up as the right arm is extended forward, until both limbs are parallel to the floor.

Hold for 10 seconds and then return to the starting position. Repeat with the opposite arm and leg and then repeat the entire sequence on each side.

4. The Supine Pelvic Tilt:

Moving on to the lumbar type exercise, this tilt works on the low back and abdominals. Lie in a neutral position on your back, with the knees bent and the feet flat on the floor. The natural curve of the lumbar spine should cause your low back to be slightly elevated off the floor. Exhale and gently pull your belly button in towards your spine, as you press your lower back into the floor. Hold for two seconds and then repeat the exercise ten times.

This exercise will improve your posture and improve lower back pain.

5. Cervical Stars:

A young looking neck is desirable as we age, and the cervical stars will give you an opportunity to work on the neck rotators, neck flexors, extensors and lateral flexors to improve range of motion and relieve neck pain.

Sit or stand keeping the neck, shoulders and torso straight, keeping the chin level look straight ahead.

Imagine there is a star in front of you with a vertical line, a horizontal line, and two diagonal lines. Trace the star shape with your head and neck by following the vertical line up and down three times. Next follow the horizontal line once, finally trace the two diagonal lines. Return to the start position and repeat five times.

Avoid hunching or tensing the shoulders and move in a slow controlled manner.

6. Thoracic Stretch:

Sit on a Swiss ball in a well -balanced neutral position with your hips directly over the center of the ball. Raise your arms and continue to extend backwards, allowing the ball to roll up your spine. If you can reach your hands to the floor then hold the position for ten seconds. To come out of the position, roll back over the ball, and bring yourself back to the sit up position.

The pectoralis, deltoids and rectus femoris muscles are worked to target the thoracic and lumber spine.

7. Leg Extension:

The quadriceps muscle is well trained by using the gym machine with weights to raise the poundage to appropriate resistance. Raise and lower the legs with a controlled movement and start with ten repetitions. The more repetitions done the tighter and harder the quadriceps will become. Your metabolism will increase with more muscle tissue in the body. The quadriceps is one of the biggest and longest muscles in the body, so it does make sense to keep this muscle in good shape.

8. Leg Curl:

The hamstrings are important muscles used in running and jumping, but unfortunately we may not be using these muscles much in our sedentary jobs. Seat yourself on the gym machine and pull down with the legs with a smooth controlled movement, working up to the weight desirable. These leg extensions and leg curls also indirectly help with abdominal muscles, as the movement continues up through the length of the body.

9. Lateral Pulldown:

The latissimus dorsi and biceps are trained in this arm exercise. Pull down on the bar until it is in front of the face and the elbows to the side of the body. This is a good exercise to prevent flabby arms which can occur in the later years of life if those arms muscles are not used. Slow pulldowns are important and increasing the reps to improve muscle tone. Do not attempt heavy weights until you get used to this exercise.

10. Fly:

This is an important exercise for women as it trains the pectoralis major or breast muscle. Grasp the handles and bring the elbows forward so that the hands meet in front of the chest. Go back to the start and do ten reps, continue to develop the muscle by increasing resistance.

11. Glute:

Rest the forearms on the arm pads and grasp the handles, and push back with the leg to work the gluteus maximus, hamstrings and quadriceps. Work both legs, starting with the lighter weights, until the muscles gain strength. This exercise will help define the buttocks and legs.

12. Row/Rear Deltoid:

The latissimus dorsi, biceps and middle trapezius, are used by pulling the weights from full extension back to the chest, bringing the elbows back to the abdomen. This is a good exercise for toning the back and shoulder muscles. Remember to keep the weights light, so that the muscles do not build into manly looking shoulders!

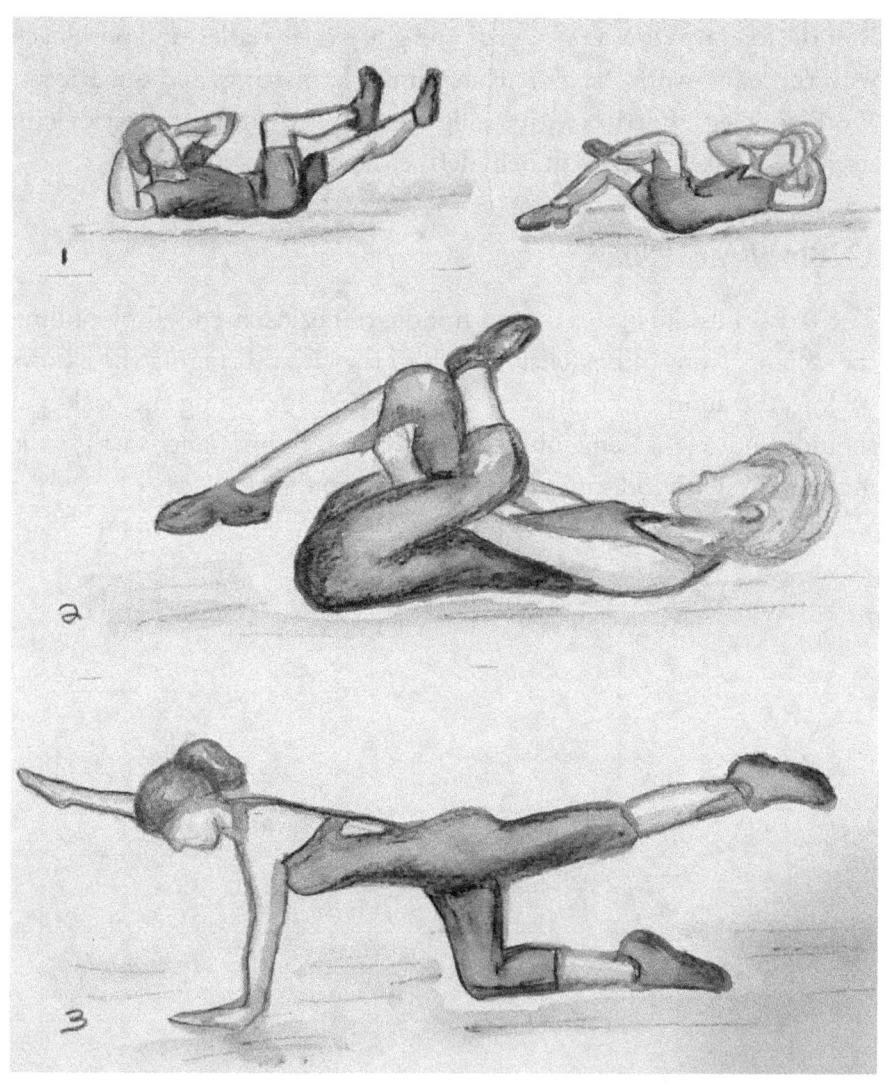

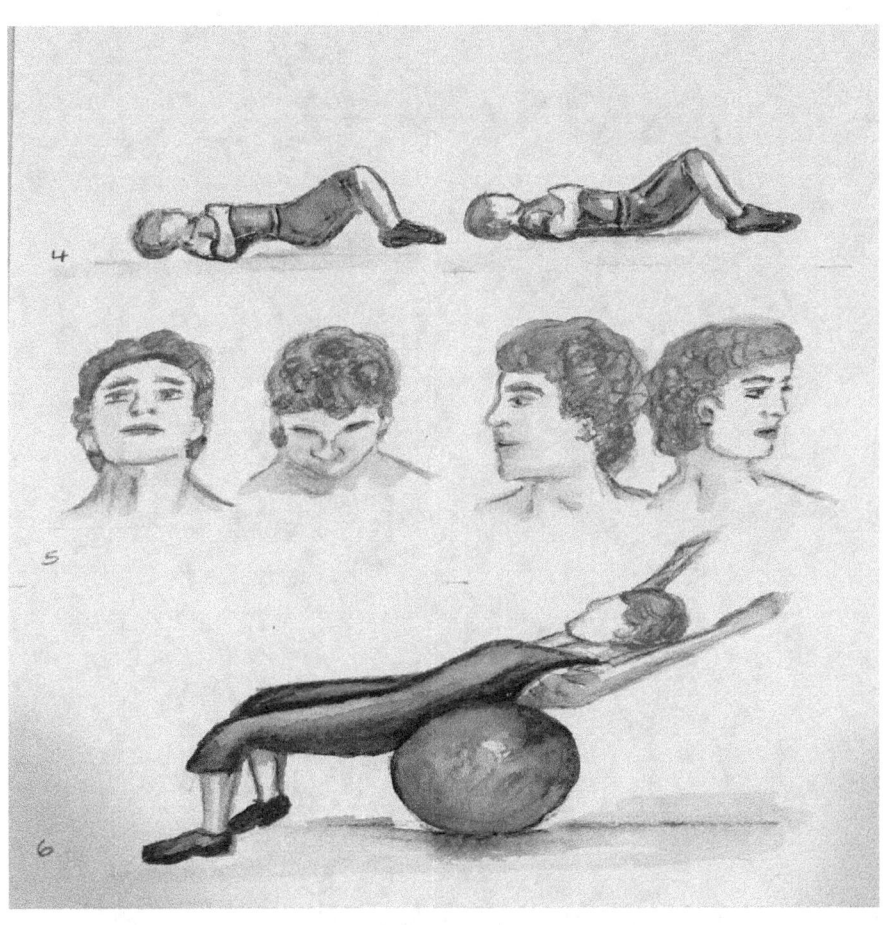

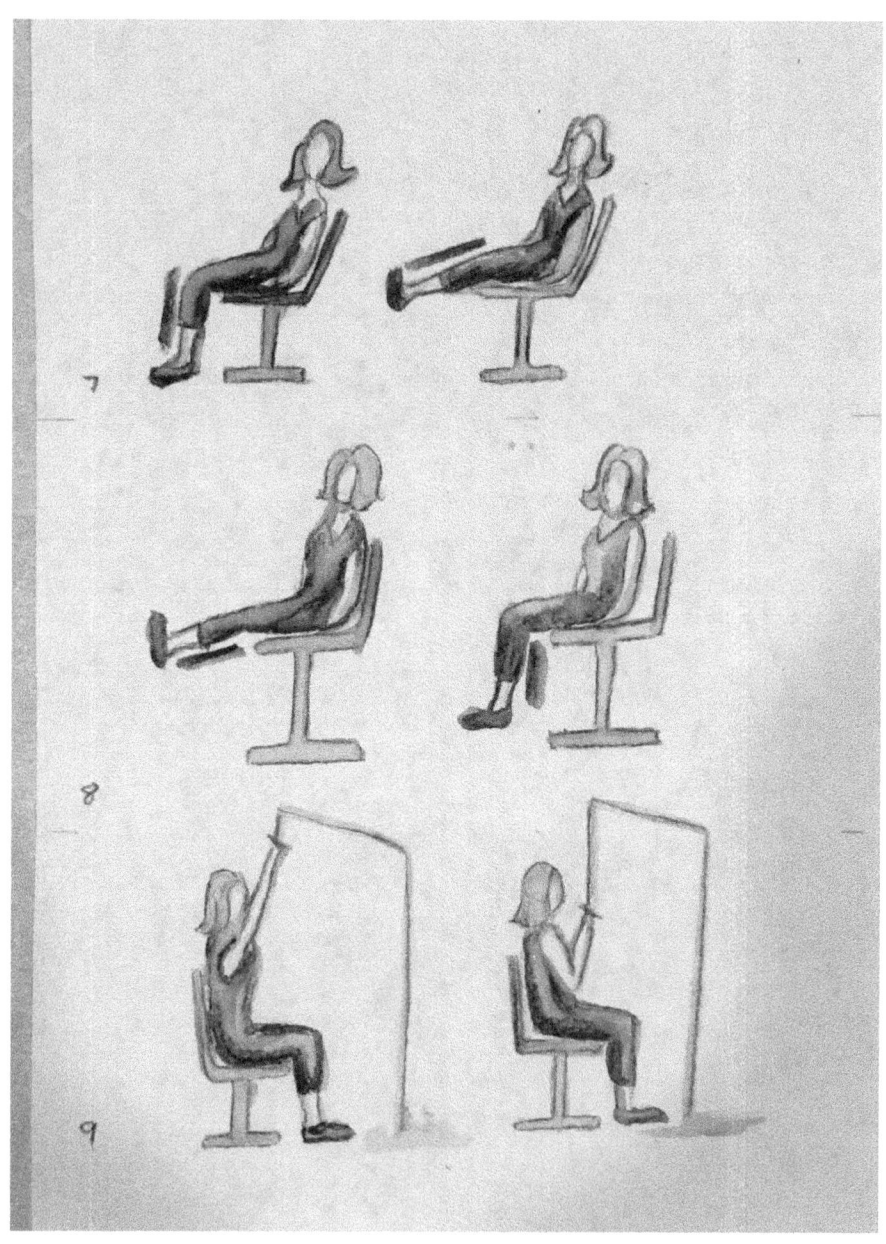

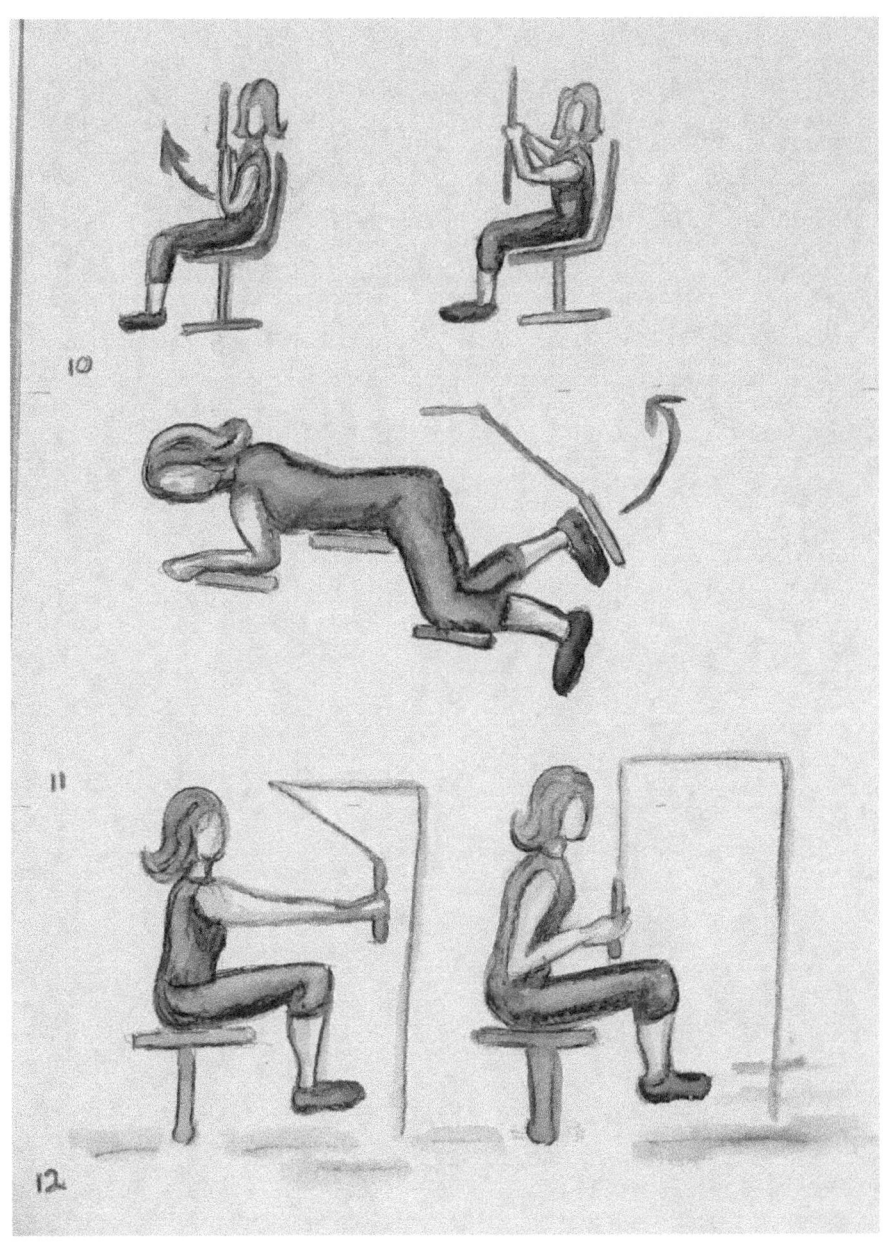

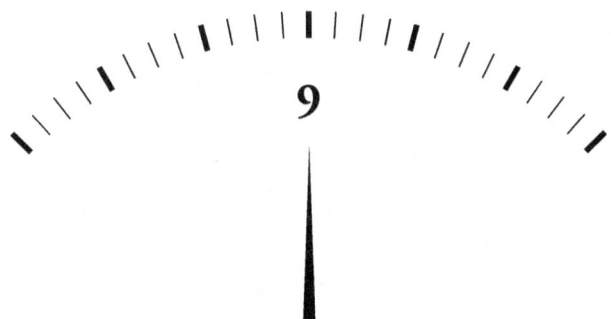

9

Dietary supplements, minerals and vitamins

It is important to obtain most of the vitamins and dietary needs from whole food consumption. On this diet, supplements are necessary, due to the decreased calorie intake. With a normal intake of calories the vitamins and minerals are absorbed and stored in the body.

There are charlatans out there who are trying to make money by claiming they have developed the elixir or pill for long life, or to cure certain nutritional ills, and this goes for weight loss pills also. Most of these claims do not work or are exaggerated, and the products are very expensive. Some of the prescriptions developed for weight loss have turned out to be dangerous and have been removed from the market, due to the FDA stepping in, after reports of adverse drug reactions. Supplements do not have to be approved by the FDA, and henceforth can be useless, toxic or worse.

Vitamins are chemical compounds necessary for growth and normal metabolism and well-being[18]. Some vitamins are essential parts of enzymes-the chemical molecules that catalyze or facilitate the completion of chemical reactions. Other vitamins form essential parts of hormones to promote and protect body health. A daily general vitamin supplement is taken on this diet to provide for these needs.

Minerals are inorganic chemical elements and participate in many biochemical and physiological processes necessary for optimal growth. If the body requires more than 100mg of a mineral each day, the substance is labelled as a mineral. If the body requires less than 100mg of the element each day the substance is labelled a trace element. Minerals that conduct electricity when dissolved in water are called electrolytes, and include sodium, potassium and chloride.

Magnesium 400mg is a required supplement on this diet, to increase bowel health. Magnesium is an important supplement that activates essential enzymes and affects metabolism of proteins and nucleic acids, and influences calcium levels inside cells. It aids muscle contractions and helps transport sodium and potassium across cell membranes. A daily multivitamin with mineral supplement is also required, containing the RDA allowance of important vitamins such as A, B, C, D, E, K and trace elements as chromium, copper and selenium.

Vitamin D levels drawn on many menopausal women may be low, even in countries where there is strong sunshine. When Vitamin D3, cholecalciferol, or vitamin D2, ergocalciferol, consumed from food or supplements enters into the general circulation, it is bound to a protein. When the vitamin is hydroxylated in the liver to 25-OH vitamin D, it then circulates in the blood for weeks. The hormone form of the vitamin is calcitriol, $1.25(OH)2$, and is active for one day. Formed in the kidney, people with chronic kidney failure take a supplement. When there is a shortage of calcium in the blood the parathyroid gland increased the production of parathyroid hormone and $1,25(OH)$ vitamin D in the kidney. Vitamin D is important in maintaining calcium balance in the blood even when dietary calcium intake is not optimal. Osteomalacia and osteoporosis can occur with inadequate Vitamin D and calcium intake, or drugs that cause malabsorption of calcium such as proton-pump inhibitor drugs and antacids.

The foods listed in this diet such as nuts, beans, cheese, eggs, peas, chicken, turkey, beef, sea food, soybeans, tuna and whole grain crackers contain such elements as phosphorus and calcium, which build strong bones and teeth and promotes energy metabolism. Iron and copper are found in chick peas, legumes, raisins, spinach, oats, soybeans and salmon.

There are many medicinal herbs with possible effects, like garlic that inhibits platelet aggregation, and helps dispose of excess fluid by increasing the amount of urine produced. These whole bulbs and roots all contain flavorings and antioxidants that are useful, such as ginger that can help with nausea and indigestion. Some informal studies have been completed on the properties and actions of medicinal herbs and chemical, but not the controlled double blind studies that have been done on FDA approved drugs. So it is hard to tell exactly how effective these agents can be, and the potency of the live or dried roots, bulbs, leaves and flowers. Some of the herbs used as supplements are ginseng, grape seed extract, kava kava, mulberry, myrrh, papaya, parsley, rose, rosemary and sage, saw palmetto, thyme and tea tree oil and willow.

Rather than trying to take supplements on an individual basis, take one multivitamin and mineral tablet daily in the morning, 1,000 to 2,000 units of vitamin D daily as well as magnesium oxide 400mg at bedtime. Fish oil 1gm may help reduce inflammation, such as arthritic pain, or hyperlipidemia.

There is also evidence that taking multiple supplements at the same time can cause overload on the absorptive carrier mechanisms, and hence will not be absorbed. These physical and chemical principals portray the intent of the engineering of our bodies. Our systems are meant to absorb small amounts of vitamins and minerals from our three small meals a day. It is not a natural way to overload our digestive tract by popping pills several times a day. There is a lot of research on vitamins and the RDA needed on each one is standard[17]. There are occasionally genomic problems which may need to be investigated by a medical doctor.

In a placebo-controlled, single-blinded cross over study, 21 healthy normocholesterolemic perimenopausal and menopausal women were assigned to receive 80mg isoflavones (plant estrogens) without soy protein for 10 weeks. Labs were taken at baseline and at the end of treatment and placebo periods. Isoflavone treatment resulted in a 26% improvement in systemic arterial compliance (arterial elasticity) compared to placebo[20]. The authors say this result compares to the same extent as achieved by HRT. Although people in certain cultures have been consuming soy foods for centuries, the efficacy and safety of concentrated isoflavones in pill form is unknown.

Soy proteins, such as soy milk, tofu and whole soy beans, are the preferred source of soy protein in the diet. Isoflavones may stimulate cancer proliferation in women with breast cancer.[21]

The information supplied above is to illustrate that there have been studies done on supplements, but a lot have not been powered with sufficient participants to produce statistically significant or reliable data. That is why medications with substantial and significant studies approved through the FDA should be the only formulations used for disease states related to vitamin and mineral deficiencies, detected by medical testing.

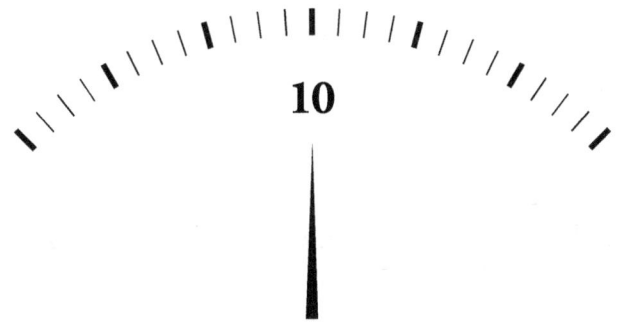

10

Recipes

The basic low calorie recipes included in the Diet cards are listed here. As mentioned previously this magical menopause diet is about whole foods, so there are very few recipes. Also a lot of busy work in the kitchen may cause more food to be available and more possibility for weight gain.

Tabouli:

One cup of parsley, either curley or Italian

2 scallions (green onions-

2 medium ripe tomatoes

One medium cucumber, most of the peel removed

1 tbsp of olive oil and 3 tbsp of fresh lemon juice

Chop the parsley, scallions and tomatoes finely, dice the cucumber, and add the dressing with salt and pepper to taste. (2 servings)

Hummus:

1 can of chick peas, drained

2 peeled garlic cloves

1 tablespoon of tahini (sesame paste)

6 tablespoons of fresh lemon juice

Salt to taste

Place the chick peas. garlic cloves, tahini, lemon juice and salt in a food processer, and process until smooth. Add extra lemon juice to correct consistency, Serving is 4 tablespoons.

Chicken Vegetable soup:

500 mls of chicken broth

Half a chopped sweet onion, sprinkled with one tablespoon of olive oil and microwaved for 2 mins

8oz of cubed, cooked chicken

10 small, chopped carrots

10 diced, celery ribs

Salt and pepper to taste

Simmer chicken broth with all ingredients added for 10 minutes. Servings=2

Mixed Bean Salad:

One can of green beans

One can of kidney beans

One can of chick peas

One can of corn

Half a diced sweet onion

One tablespoon of olive oil, one tablespoon of agave syrup or honey, one tablespoon of rice vinegar, salt and pepper to taste

Mix all ingredients together and refrigerate. 8 servings

(pinto beans can be substituted for kidney beans)

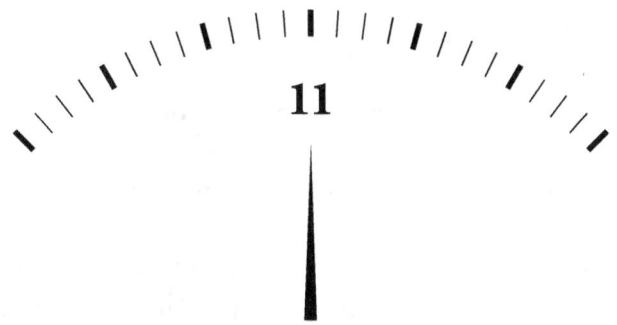

11

Diet Stories

1: Bulemia

JM ran into the bathroom and locked the door. She pulled up the toilet seat and leaned over so that her face was close to the bowl. She stuck her index and middle finger down her throat and started to vomit. The orange liquid race dup through her throat and spewed into the toilet, and the chunks of hamburger sank to the bottom while the partially dissolved French fries floated on top. She grabbed some toilet tissue and mopped at her mouth. Her stomach felt empty again, the sick feeling receded, and relief flooded her head.

She flushed the toilet and rinsed her mouth with cold water, and swallowed to relieve the acid in her throat. Her baby blue eyes stared back at her from the mirror, tearing from the effort. Her twenty two year old waistline could only have measured twenty four inches at most, and the washed out size 4 blue jeans hugged her hips.

JM returned to her friends still sitting under the pine trees, finishing their fast food lunch. The other two girls did not look up, but kept on in earnest conversation. What topic would be on the math test on Wednesday?

JM opened her text book and started on an integration problem.

"What answer did you get for 2C?" she asked.

"Oh, I haven't started that exercise", the blonde girl responded.

"Aren't you nervous you won't finish by tomorrow? Jessica said.

"No, I have all tonight to go over it", the other girl said. "I think I'll go back to the dorm and take a nap. "All this food has made me sleepy".

JM was in her last year of college and the math final over tomorrow, she would only have the biology exam left to sit on Friday.

She wanted to be a school teacher and would be heading back to Los Angeles in the fall, to start substitute teaching in the high schools. Her boyfriend was also graduating with a bioengineering degree and they planned on finding an apartment together.

JM loved Todd so much and was excited about their future together. After all JM's dad was an engineer and he and Todd had discussed possible employment at his firm. Todd has let JM know how important a good physical shape was to him, working out at the university gym daily, lifting weights until his biceps were bulging. He took pleasure in circling his hands around her waist and squeezing, and then laughing about how small it was.

Todd even went so far as to day that he could date no one else, because he loved her small size so much. He was critical of heavier girls, and always complimented JM on her physical attributes. One day at a Thanksgiving dinner at her parents, he had made fun of her, on the side, saying that she looked like a stuffed turkey, as her stomach was distended. That was when she had learned to relieve herself in the method she was accustomed to now. She so much preferred to hear Todd admiring her waistline, and being able to fit into her tight size 4 jeans. She even threw up after eating four chocolate chip cookies and a glass of milk. Anytime she thought the calories would add up to cause weight gain, she would actually consume more, then drink liquid and evacuate her stomach.

Once, when visiting home, her mother had inquired why the toilet had orange particles around the rim, but Jessica had an answer for that. She solved the problem by letting her mother know that she had the stomach flu, and there was no more discussion on the subject.

Jessica's eating habits had changed while at college and she either nibbled or ate nothing, or she consumed all she wanted, knowing she would not take the calorie consequences. She had noticed that her teeth had begun to feel sensitive, and she had pain in the lower left molar. The dentist had said she would need a root canal.

Her hands had also turned orange due to damaging her liver, from near starvation on occasions. Somehow her disease was not noticed by family or friends. Everyone thought it was normal to eat so much and be so thin.

2: Anorexia:

ST had an hour glass figure. She stood five feet five inches tall and had perfect skin. Her eyes were a pale aquamarine blue and the black pupils were prominent.

ST's mother, Mildred, also had an hour glass figure, which she regained quickly after ST, her only child, was born.

The girls, as they referred to themselves, ate very lightly, while Sean, Mildred's husband, was absent on overseas business trips. Sean was a software salesman as well as a biological engineer.

ST left the ranch style home at 7:15am every morning to reach Mt Pleasant high school in time for assembly at 8am. She rode her red bike up the hill, pedaling hard to reach the top. She had not eaten any breakfast, so she was accessing stored glycogen from her liver. The girls had not eaten much dinner the previous night, just some carrot sticks and hummus dip with a few pita chips. Mildred had not provided a school lunch for ST either. It was her long day on Monday. While the other girls ate their peanut butter and jelly sandwiches, Jeanine sat and looked on.

She could feel one of her migraine headaches coming on in Math class, the aura presenting with bright lights flashing in dots and zig zags across her field of vision. She felt dizzy and sick, and as the pulsating headache began, she left for the domestic science classroom, where the sick room was located. The kindly domestic science matron called Mildred to come and pick ST up.

When ST was back in her bedroom she lay down in the darkened room. She was hypoglycemic, but she knew there was no food in the refrigerator. She took her paracetamol and fell asleep.

The next morning ST ate a slice of toast with margarine and jelly, before she left for school. She was feeling better after the nights rest and Sean was back in town, so he dropped her off. Mildred handed her a peanut butter and jelly sandwich, as well as a large, red apple, as she exited with her father.

ST had finished her classes at 2pm and Sean was on time to pick her up.

"Mom is cooking us spaghetti Bolognese for dinner" he smiled at her, as she jumped into the Mercedes.

"Oh, that is my favorite meal!" ST laughed.

She had field hockey practice at 4pm through 5:30pm and after that they sat down as a family to enjoy the dinner.

"I bought this hamburger meat on special", she informed them, as she dished out a generous helping for Sean. The pasta was cooked al dente and the well browned meat with spices and tomato sauce tasted delicious. Mildred served herself a very small amount of meat and a few strands of spaghetti on her plate. ST followed suite, with a similar small portion.

Sean was well covered, but not fat, and enjoyed his meal. Glancing at the girls, he noted,

"Oh I suppose you girls are watching your weight! I'll finish up the bolognese."

Mildred has added steamed green peas as a side dish, and he finished these too.

Mildred was a homemaker and did not work out of the house. She managed on what Sean gave her for house-keeping and stuck religiously to her budget. She also kept some of the budget money to buy clothes and make up to show off her beautiful figure and face.

ST did not complain about the lack of food in the house while Sean was away. She accepted her mother's custom of missing meals, and in fact had become anorexic herself. She had been invited to some of her friend's houses for meals and was surprised to see how much food was stored in the refrigerator, and the constant munching going on. Some of the friends were much heavier than she was, so she soon realized that was because they ate three or more times what she did in a day.

When she had the "flu and the mother had taken her to Dr. Brown's office, he had commented on her weight.

"ST weighs 105 pounds", he looked up at Mildred.

"Well I am only 118 pounds", she replied, smiling.

"At this stage of development, it would be better for Jeanine to weigh 125 pounds for her height and build" Dr. Brown explained.

"She plays in the field hockey team" Mildred stated. "ST is one of the best goal shooters" she added.

"Yes, but for an eighteen year old she should have more muscle" Dr. Brown continued, "are you feeding her meals with proteins such as meat, chicken, beans, cheese and nuts?"

"We had spaghetti Bolognese this week" she said, "and roast chicken also."

"Well she may need larger portions of food, and more frequent meals" Dr. Brown finished.

Parents of her friends had tried to fatten her up, offering snacks such as potato chips, candy or even burgers, but she mostly refused. She had become like her mother, Mildred, comfortable with watching while others ate. As her mother said, there was always peanut butter and jelly to make a sandwich.

3. The Closet Eater:

TD removed her salad from the refrigerator. Two cups of shredded lettuce, one tomato and one small cucumber, and three ounces of chicken breast were packed into the plastic container. She measured two tablespoons of low calorie ginger dressing and drizzled the dressing over the salad.

"Is that all you're going to eat?" Tracy asked. Tracy was her co-worked at the bank, and they had taken a break together.

"Yes," TD replied. "I am watching my weight." TD looked down at her waistline, and her stomach protruded. The last time she had weighed herself was months ago, but she suspected she was still in the 160's, too heavy for her 5ft 3 inch height and medium frame.

Tracy had a 6 inch sandwich filled with cold cuts. "This is really all I eat in the day," she said.

"Food is too expensive to buy more, and I don't keep much in my apartment."

"All I know", TD replied "Is that food just goes stale, if you don't finish it all. Even with the yoghurt I buy, the expiration date comes up fast".

TD thought about the supply of food in her pantry at home. She always bought potato chips, cookies and candy when she went grocery shopping, just to tide her over if she didn't feel like heating something up.

"You always eat salads", Tracy observed.

"Do you have a problem with metabolism? That salad can't have many calories".

"I think I need to exercise more" TD replied, avoiding the calorie question. "It's just when I get home, I feel so tired I just curl up in front of the TV."

She lived alone in a one bedroom apartment, 2 blocks from the bank. She had watched her favorite sitcom last evening, and had opened a favorite bag of salt and vinegar chips. She had bought a large bag on sale and felt happy she had cashed in on a bargain. She loved the sour taste of the vinegar and the crunch as she bit into the chip. The crunching and nibbling had gone on through most of the hour long sitcom. She knew the labelling showed ten servings, and 150 calories per serving, but she felt she deserved to eat what she wanted after a long day at work. She felt full and had tossed the empty bag into the trash and had made her salad for lunch the following day.

She had a box of chocolates as well as red vines and coconut cookies left for the rest of the week.

She never took those items into the bank, as the other workers felt entitled to help themselves, and very little was left for TD. Leaving those tasty items in the closet at home, meant she would enjoy the full benefit herself. Her serotonin levels were soaring and she had slept soundly.

"That salad probably does not fill you up", Tracy said. "Do you eat a lot when you go home?"

"No", TD replied," Just a few potato chips."

"I have heard 14 hours fasting is effective" Tracy stated. "My Mother started that last year and she dropped twenty pounds."

TD went home to enjoy another sitcom evening at home. As the raucous laughter of the background audience echoed in her ears, she reached for favorite box of chocolates. Her very favorite was the almond brittle, the nutty, buttery flavors lingered in her mouth, giving a feeling of pleasure. Next she tried the dark, chocolate ganache, rich and creamy, a taste that relaxed her. The caramel covered in milk chocolate was chewy, the cherry cordial was sweet and tart at the same time. Her blood sugar level crept up with each bite, but she had to taste just one more, until the box of 15 chocolates was consumed, not one left. The calorie information was on the box, but per gram, and she could not make heads or tails out of it.

TD brushed her teeth well, before falling into a sugar coma.

4. Gluttony:

AL was parked outside MG's Donut Store. He ordered his usual, 2 glazed cake donuts, and 2 chocolate frosted, fried donuts. He ate all four pieces and washed them down with piping hot coffee.

It was a typical, sunny day in Southern California, seventy degrees with a few white clouds floating in the bright, blue sky. AL sat in his Toyota Prius, proud to be driving a hybrid vehicle, and saving the planet.

The donut habit had started in Chicago, in the subzero winter, when AL had passed by the donut store on the way to work daily. The sugar from the first donut had helped with the early morning blues, and a second donut had started the serotonin upswing. He was also enticed by the many varieties of donuts, and sometimes his impulsive food cravings directed him to purchase 3 or 4 types. The combination of coffee and donut seemed to give AL endless energy. AL was in his mid-forties, and transferred from Chicago to California to sell insurance. He was obese, being twenty percent over his ideal body weight. He had noticed that people in California were more interested in physical appearance, and body bulk could not be hidden under winter coats. He calculated it may have something to do with the year round sunshine and temperate weather.

Most of his clients refused the donut when offered. These were the same people who visited a gym several times a week, and drank iced vert green teas, instead of coffee.

His doctor had told him he needed to lose weight, at his annual physical and wellness visit, last May. He let him know he was at higher risk for heart attack and stroke, with his combined comorbidity of high blood pressure and obesity. The appointment had only lasted fifteen minutes with the physician, who then left to rush into the next patient, and although Archie had been alarmed at first, the visit now receded into the back of his memory.

When lunch time arrived, AL made a run for the nearest fast food joint, for a burger, fries and soda. He had continued this habit since high school days, when he had been a growing boy, and needed the 1,000 calories for lunch. Nowadays the burger sat in his stomach, and sometimes he thought he had esophageal reflux. Pepcid or Zantac OTC seemed to relieve the pressure. The burger and fries tasted good, with the oily and salty flavors, but he was starting to realize that the fast food was not good for his digestion. He thought that he should try one of the salads, containing only 300 calories a serving, but he just felt he was paying for rabbit food! His wife had suggested yoghurt along with the salad, to provide a protein boost, but he had never eaten yoghurt and was not about to start anytime soon.

When AL arrived home from work, his wife had a well- balanced meal waiting for him. She was a good cook, and unlike most other women, she did not like to save left overs. The balance was left in the kitchen, until AL went in to do the washing up. He would have a few spoons of his favorites, and then toss the balance. His wife skipped breakfast, and took non-fat Greek yoghurt for lunch, so her main meal of the day was dinner. She skipped desert, but made sure that a stock of ice-cream, and cookies, was available for AL, who had a sweet tooth. After washing up, AL would settle in front of the TV, with a bowl of ice-cream, and several cookies. He called it his feel good dessert, and could feel the calming effect, after his heavy caseload of the day, and sometimes irate clients.

"Thank-you dear", he called to his wife, "that was a great dinner", as he reached for one last cookie, before turning in for the night.

5. The Healthy Eater:

LA was preparing her fruit salad for breakfast in a large bowl. She added one banana, an apple, and an orange, all chopped together, and she knew the orange juice would keep the banana fresh. Then she prepared 2 hard- boiled eggs to provide the protein, to support the fiber and antioxidants in her fruit salad.

She had consumed her dinner of grilled salmon and broccoli, with half a baked potato. She had eaten the full 8oz piece of salmon, because it contained omega oils, as well as the proteins that are good for her. Then she had needed something sweet, after all the fish oils. She ate half a cup of toasted coconut and a handful of dark chocolate cherries. As her nightcap she drank 8oz of almond milk. Her private trainer had asked her to consume at least 200gms of protein a day to keep her muscles toned

She had eaten a double burger for lunch with cheese, no fries, and a diet cola, as sugar was not included in her regimen. She was happy with her 120gms of protein and planned on adding another 50gms with her protein shake. Her trainer had not told her to bother counting calories, although she was eating over 2,500/day.

She was preparing for a boxing tournament and needed to be in peak performance and was currently weighing in at 160lbs, and had to lose 6 pounds to be in the under 155 lb. category.

LA was as strong as she had been in several years, and expected to win the contest. The only problem is she could not shed the last 5 pounds, her trainer had told her that she needed to maintain the healthy diet for her strength.

Her MD had told her to consume fewer calories, and she would drop the weight, but when she reduced the proteins her muscles lost strength, and her concentration waned. If she reduced her carbs then her mental moves were slower.

She tried eating only salad and proteins, but found she had lost her strength and quick movements, and then she found a book that contained a diet showing much less protein, but with the same amount of carbs she was currently eating. She found that by adding 2 protein shakes a day, she was up to her 120gms of protein, but with fewer calories.

Her day to box came and she was excited to get her match over with, she was just at 154.5 pounds and in peak condition. Her coach had trained her well and she won the match!

After the match LA was careful to continue with her daily routine of running and jump rope, as well as weight training, so not to gain any weight back. She kept a strict regimen of weighing herself naked every morning, and never missed a weigh in!

References

1. Atkins for Life. Robert C Atkins MD
2. Prevention Healthy Cooking. Retting Newman, RD, David Joachim.
3. Fit not Fat at Forty. Rodale Books
4. Eat and Heal. Editors of F, C and A Medical Publishing
5. A review on the effect of diet on cardiovascular calcification: Rachel Nicholl, John McLaren Howard et al.
6. Healthy Back Anatomy. Phillip Striano, DC.
7. Eat Right for your Type. Dr. P J D'Adamo.
8. South Beach Diet. Arthur Agatston MD
9. Lose Weight the Smart Lo Carb Way.
10. Nature's Prescriptions- Foods, Vitamins and Supplements that prevent disease. FC and A Medical Publishing.
11. What to Eat When. Michael F. Roizen, M.D, Michael Crupain, M.D., MPH.
12. New Year, New Diet. Dr. Ken Fujioka, Director of Nutrition and Metabolic Research, Scripps Clinic.
13. Isaiah 58 Holy Bible
14. Treatment of Symptoms of the Menopause. An Endocrine Society Clinical Practice Guideline. Stuenkel, C.A., Davis, S, R.,et al, J of Clinical Endocrinology and Metabolism, November 1, 2015 vol 100, Issue 11

15. Role of Hormone Therapy in the Management of Menopause. Shifren, Schiff I. Obstet. Gynecol. 2010, 115 (4); 839-855.

16. North American Menopause Society. The 2012 hormone therapy position statement. Menopause 2012.19.(3) 257-273

17. Perspectives in Nutrition; Gordon, M, Wardlow, Jeff. 7th Edition McGraw Hill.

18. Vitamins, herbs and Minerals, The complete Guide. H.Winter Griffith, M.D.

19. The Health Professional's Guide to Popular Dietary Supplements. Allison Sarubin MS, RD.

20. Nestel PJ, Yamashita T, Pomeroy S, et al. Soy isoflavones improve systemic arterial compliance but not plasma lipids in menopausal and perimenopausal women. Arterioscle. Throm. Vasc Biol 1997:17:3392-3398

21. McMichael-Phillips DF, Harding C, Morton M, et al. Effects of soy protein supplementation on epithelial proliferation in the histologically normal human breast. Am J Clin Nutr 1998:68:14315-14355.

22. Mackenzie Moritz, Emily Knezevitch, et al Updates in the Treatment of Postmenopausal Osteoporosis: US Pharmacist Sept.2019

About the Author

The Magical Menopause Diet is written from a personal experience as well as a scientific standpoint. The author is a pharmacist with knowledge of menopausal experiences and medications that can be used to alleviate menopausal symptoms. Weight gain during the menopause was a problem for the author, so a diet was devised that would work to reduce caloric intake. Mary Douzjian was successful at losing 25 pounds over an 8 month period and keeping the weight off. She wanted to share this information with readers who have been struggling with weight loss, as well as highlight certain disease states that may be caused by increase weight gain over the years spent in menopause. Mary Douzjian has over 35 years of experience in the medical field and enjoys analyzing medical information for the consumer.